Extraordinary Healing
Ordinary Miracle

Extraordinary
Healing
Ordinary
Miracle

Choosing WellBeing Over Fighting Cancer

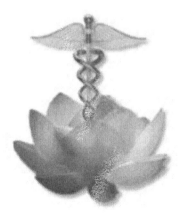

Patricia French Crilly, R.N.

Library of Congress Control Number: 2015910833
IBSN: 978-0-9965668-0-3

Cover Design by Kim Sillen
Edited by Christie Stratos, Proof Positive
Author photograph by Joe Peoples
Book interior design by Jean Boles

To all Holistic and Alternative Healing Arts Practitioners who so selflessly share their gift of compassionate healing to relieve pain and suffering of the mind, body, and spirit. You push ego aside with the knowing that all healing comes not by you but through you to light the path of joyful ease and comfort to those whom you are of service.

The soul always knows what to do to heal itself.
The challenge is to silence the mind.

- Caroline Myss

CONTENTS

FOREWORD

S tart here first!
If you or someone you know has been diagnosed with cancer, you have to start with this book first.

You'll meet Patricia French Crilly, a charmingly sarcastic and witty RN, who after learning she had invasive ovarian cancer, created her own healing odyssey to fully reclaim her WellBeing despite an ominous prognosis.

I met Nurse Crilly at a marketing conference in May of 2013. It was one of those synchronistic events...I was at a meeting in Chicago, heard of this event, and was invited as a guest. Pat stood up to introduce herself. Not only was she a nurse but a practitioner of several modalities in the holistic and alternative healing arts. She wanted to share her healing story and talked about her desire to write a book to impart how she was able to get past the fear.

Get past the fear?? How do you get past the fear of the big "C"?

I was fascinated!

As an entrepreneurial consultant and advisor specializing in integrative healthcare practitioners, I wanted to learn more about her story. Soon after, I became her coach and we started talking once a week, and Pat started writing. Every chapter she shared with me brought me deeper into her odyssey. She was a patient who happened to be a nurse and she saw the healthcare system from a unique point of view. She's feisty but compassionate and even though was as vulnerable as any patient would be, she questioned and sought answers and emblazed a path different than most. I was always captivated by each example and interaction she had. And I learned from her too.

In the two years that we have worked together, I have found her to be incredibly funny, clever and someone who has an insatiable desire to share her message: overcoming the fear, altering self-limiting beliefs and focusing on WellBeing catapulting the patient into a new way of 'being' about a cancer. Actually, any disease. It's her 'Healing Triad'.

Extraordinary Healing, Ordinary Miracle: Choosing WellBeing Over Fighting Cancer offers you a new perspective on healing. Read on and meet Pat. She'll make you laugh, and sometimes I bet you'll cry. You'll learn from her story while she empowers and inspires you on your own healing journey.

Live well,

Evie M. Caprel, BA, CHTP

PREFACE

There are more than twelve hundred book titles listed on Amazon that were written for, by or about cancer survivors. Many are compilations of inspiring personal stories of survival or of those extolling the benefits of diet, nutrition or exercise as the answer for cancer. Others offer scholarly allopathic treatment options alongside a host of holistic, natural, spiritual, religious, and energy healing to name but a few. There are, of course, an assortment of full-on quackery, snake oil cures and conspiracy theories insisting that a cure for every kind of cancer exists and is being withheld by a greedy few. Many books include an endless and dizzying combination of all of the afore-mentioned possible avenues to explore for those newly diagnosed with cancer.

I certainly have not read them all. Only two or three in truth. I did, however, read the overviews and reviews of a hundred or so. And now here I am adding my own book to this already crowded arena. What made me think that this well-represented field needed yet another cancer book?

My story of healing cancer, though apparently rare, is not unique. I share many similarities with others who have recovered their WellBeing after cancer. Where I parted ways most significantly was in completely changing my language around cancer. I eschewed the conventional vernacular that is so prevalent in the cancer lexicon. Some have said that it is just a matter of semantics, citing that if you say to*may*to and I say to*mah*to, it is still a tomato. True enough, however, there is great power in words. Your words spoken or unspoken express your thoughts and as Mike Dooley, author of *Infinite Possibilities* says, "Thoughts become things; choose them wisely."

You will see many such examples in the following pages. I do not try to foist any of my cancer language quirks upon anyone. Take them or leave them. Embrace them if they resonate with you or toss them aside. In the above paragraphs, while not exactly changing any common cancer lingo, I have skirted around it. Specifically, "My story of healing" and "recovered WellBeing after cancer" replaces the more frequently used phrase, "The story of surviving *my* cancer..."

Don't see the difference? I focused on creating an environment of healing my body so that the cancer could not flourish rather than seeking to be cured of the cancer. I also did not take ownership of the disease. It was not *my* cancer. Perhaps you noticed my use of the oddly spelled "WellBeing". This one is a biggie for me. WellBeing, in my humble opinion, is far greater than wellness being the absence of illness. I believe that it is an absolute state of being in balance and harmony of the mind, body and spirit. Am I always in that state of being? Not even most of the time, however, that is what I strive toward. I am, as we all are, a work in progress.

The last bit about language that I want to mention is one that has greatly upset some people and has also given a new and empowering perspective to many others with whom I have shared my story. I want to go a little more in depth with this idea because I believe it was at the crux of how I viewed everything about cancer and WellBeing.

A term you will never hear me use about myself is "cancer survivor". It is not a moniker that I ever warmed up to. I prefer to think that the cancer did not survive me. I chose not to take on the role of victim. We have all been victimized at one time or another in our lives. By that, I mean being controlled or manipulated physically, emotionally and/or spiritually by another person or organization. Cancer can do that. It can render you completely powerless. It can paralyze you with fear...if you let it. We've all been taught to fear cancer. We have been enculturated to allow ourselves to be held hostage by the mere threat or possibility of cancer. How often have we heard the hushed whispers about one who has fallen victim to the big "C"? So powerful and fearsome is this disease that we dare not speak its name.

I did not give cancer any such power. I did not fight the cancer. I did not battle the cancer. I did not vow to beat the cancer. I made no declaration of war on the cancer. Fight, battle, beat and war are words we use when we are pushing against something; of being in opposition. I wondered how one, actually, fights cancer. How does one do battle with cancer? If I had put my thoughts and energy into fighting cancer, I could not have put my thoughts and energy into being well. Fighting takes a lot of effort, strength and energy. As Michael Jackson said, "I'm a lover, not a fighter." I chose to use my energy for healing. I chose to raise the vibration of my energy and use it to invite healing in rather than push cancer out. The fact is that I never really thought of myself as "sick". The cancer became a part of my body so declaring war on it would be tantamount to declaring war on myself. I had no desire for my body to become a battleground with cancer treatment leaving a swath of destruction in its path.

Mother Theresa was asked if she would join a march *against* war. She declined saying she would happily march *for* peace. One might ask, "What is the difference?" Pushing against war focuses energy on the violence, brutality and tyranny that are the means of the oppressors to justify their end. Protesting these tactics is counterproductive for peace because it continues to shine its light on the negativity. This may sound naive to believe that focusing on allowing love, harmony and cooperation to flow will, ultimately, lead to peace by default.

So it is with cancer. Not pushing against it allows healing energy to flow. I know that being locked in a battle with cancer has always been in our vernacular. Those who won that battle proudly proclaim survivor status which is fine; however, what do we then call those who do not win their battle with cancer? Losers? Certainly not! I call them the bravest of the brave.

Many believe that cancer is a mortal enemy; a foe to be reckoned with and would vehemently disagree with me when I say that cancer is a victimless disease which holds no tangible power over us.

I have heard people say that they made friends with their cancer. Others have chosen to love their cancer and to thank it for the lessons it taught them. This certainly puts a positive spin on things; however, to me it still feels like giving up your power to a group of cells that have run amuck. I chose to create a belief about cancer that dovetailed with my overall philosophy of life and my spiritual leanings. My intention is not to disparage those who choose to kill the cancer or love it to death or even to declare themselves survivors. It is all about whatever works to get you through it. In looking back, the language I learned from my parents' fearful conversation about a neighbor battling cancer or the medical speak I learned in nursing school did not serve me well. This book offers an alternative perspective that I found helpful and may certainly be of help to others. When people say with respect and admiration that I fought cancer and beat it, I politely explain that I was never a victim locked in battle with a mighty foe, so please, don't call me a cancer survivor. So what do I call myself if not a survivor? I call myself an Extraordinary Healer.

In Part I, the chronology of my healing odyssey unfolds in real time and in Part II, I deconstruct how my healing came about. I discovered some surprising insights along the way. I never fully dissected my healing in any great detail before I began to write this book. What I learned in retrospect was that there were three things that stood out as crucial to the outcome which I share in considerable depth throughout this book. I call them my Healing Triad. First and foremost I needed to overcome the fear that at first came in like a tsunami followed by some powerful aftershocks in a crescendo of fear. At other times it crept in insidiously. Sometimes that was the hardest to deal with because I never saw it coming until I was already in its mighty grip.

The second challenge was to completely overhaul my belief system. I had a long-held belief that cancer was a death sentence and that unimaginable pain and suffering was inevitable. The third discovery was that I needed to take back my power. Some of my power was taken from me by a well-intentioned albeit paternalistic healthcare system and some I gave away. At times I did this willingly and at others unwittingly. This was by far the most difficult hurdle to overcome. How I long for the day when the doctor's, first words to a patient are, "We will work together using what medicine has to offer and the power of your mind, body and spirit to restore your WellBeing."

Certainly, there were other factors that led to my healing, as evidenced by the commonalities I shared with the many cases of extraordinary healing which have been well documented by Kelly Turner, Ph.D. in her inspiring book, *Radical Remission*. The many aspects of my own healing each aligned with the three points of my Healing Triad.

In the interest of full disclosure, I explored any and every avenue that I needed for complete healing and recovery of my WellBeing, from integrating conventional medicine with the holistic and alternative healing arts to the downright woo-woo. The bottom line is that what I did worked for me and that's all that really mattered to me.

If you or a loved one is dealing with cancer, no matter where you are in the course of the disease, I hope that you will find within these pages even a morsel of inspiration, hope and courage. I truly believe that as long as you draw breath, everyday ordinary miracles make extraordinary healing possible.

Be well,

Nurse Crilly

ACKNOWLEDGEMENTS

I am so blessed that I was able to stick around to express my gratitude for the serendipitous synchronicity of events that led to my extraordinary healing. Although my intention was clear from the get go, the path to reclaiming my WellBeing was unerringly revealed to me with each tentative step. In addition to being thankful for the sometimes obscure and occasionally neon lit sign posts along the way, are some individuals who deserve special recognition for their role in getting me from there to here.

In order of appearance, the founding members of my personal Wellbeing Pep Squad are Lois Brown, Sue "Snordie" Nordemo, Roxy Cortese and Doris Cruz. Each one supported my desire, intention and ultimately my belief that complete healing was possible, indeed, doable with unconditional and unwavering love and cheers at every turn. You all have my eternal gratitude.

To the Mooney/Decker clan, my big Irish family through affection, who are always there, no matter what even when they don't know they are "being there". To you, I say "Thank you! Or as our Gaelic ancestors would say, "Go raibh maith agat!"

Pat Evans (aka "The Other Pat"), my BFF and sister in the true essence of the word, kept me on an even keel no matter how rough the tide. Thank you, thank you and thank you again! I am also thankful that you didn't have to find a new BFF.

My baby sister, Jean, really stepped up to the plate despite her own health challenges and is a daily reminder of what family truly is. Thanks sister girl.

Special thanks to Dr. Cleary, my hematologist who unraveled the mystery of my symptoms. You are a true life saver.

Gynormous props to Dr. Grace, who gave me the space for me to be me. Your kindness, compassion and skill as a surgeon was a medical trifecta. Thank you just doesn't seem adequate to express my undying (quite literally) gratitude. Oh and thanks too for cutting around my belly button and not through it (*yuck!*). I really appreciate that.

There are so many others who contributed to my ultimate healing and I hope that I have thanked you adequately along the way. If I have not, I am sorry. Just know that I am grateful to you all.

I have thanked all of those kind souls who helped to get me from there to here and it is their collective support that allowed me to be in a position now to share my healing odyssey with you.

Lastly, I owe a debt of gratitude to Evie Caprel, my friend and mentor for making this book possible. Without her support, guidance and persistent yet gentle nudging, I would still be telling you all that I am going to write a book about my experience...probably...soon...someday. You helped me make what seemed to be an impossible task possible. Thank you for being my literary doula.

PROLOGUE

The story that you will read in the body of this book actually begins here. I had to go back an entire year for you to truly appreciate my story as it unfolded.

Got Clots?
April 27, 2008

I stopped at the grocery store to pick up a few things on my way home from work. As I left the store, I looked up at the clear blue sky and was filled with a sense of peaceful WellBeing. I opened the passenger side of my car to put the groceries in when suddenly I tripped, seemingly over thin air. My right foot did a very slight side-to-side wibble-wobble as I lunged into the front seat of the car in an effort to spare my right elbow, knee and ankle from injury as they had already taken a beating over the years from sports and, I have to admit, some clumsiness. I looked to see what could have caused me to trip and I saw no impediment except for a little wee stone wedged into the gap where the two concrete sections of the curb met. The funny thing (really not so funny as it turned out) is that I felt a little "pop" in my right foot followed by some vague discomfort. Just walk it off, I thought, as I congratulated myself on the great save to my right appendages and then headed home.

During the evening, I had all but forgotten about my little mishap. Leaving for work the following morning, my right foot felt a little strange. Not exactly painful but a little weak and unstable. At the time, I was caring for a young man who was ventilator dependent and confined to a wheelchair. I would meet him at his home in the morning, take the bus to school with him and accompany him as he went to his classes. I attended to his needs throughout the day and then took the bus home with him in the afternoon. The work was not very physically demanding, but it was a huge school and while he tooled around in his electric wheelchair, I had to schlep along behind him. An interesting side note was that by attending school with him, I was re-experiencing junior and senior year some thirty years later. As a Baby Boomer, it was a little disconcerting to have had such vivid and personal memories of what the students now considered ancient history.

My foot was becoming increasingly achy as the day progressed. At home, I removed my shoes and I noticed that the top of my right foot was slightly swollen and getting a little black and blue. *Humph. What's that about?* By the third day, I was having significant pain when walking and the bruising was up to my ankle, although the swelling was still minimal. I decided that I needed some type of support for my foot. It wasn't my ankle that was the problem, so an ankle support was not the answer. I didn't have heel spurs or bunions or hammertoes. What I had was pain in the middle section of my foot, so I Googled pain in the mid foot and what popped up took me by surprise.

Each listing for mid foot pain described an injury to the Lis Franc ligament. That is the ligament that goes across the top of the foot and holds the bones from your toes to your ankle in alignment. A severe tear can cause those bones to crumple like pickup sticks. The warning to stay off the injured foot and seek medical attention immediately was included in every listing. Ignoring this advice while continuing to bear weight on the injured foot could lead to devastating and permanent disability.

I dug out a pair of crutches from an old knee injury and went to a Doc-in-a-Box (a walk-in urgent care center). An x-ray was taken and I was assured that no fracture was evident. I told the doc that I was pretty sure it was a Lis Franc injury. He told me that I did not have enough swelling for it to be that kind of injury. Here's the thing: injuries don't swell much on me. He told me to keep off it for a week or so and ice it.

I asked the doctor for a walking boot (that's what Google said to ask for) and he suggested that I get a Dr. Scholl's ankle support. *It is NOT my ankle, you numbskull!* Okay, by now I was experiencing some pretty severe pain and the doc said to take Motrin (which had not helped thus far) because he didn't think I needed anything stronger. I asked for a referral to an orthopedic doctor or a podiatrist. Perhaps in a week or two if it was no better.

This doc poo-pooed everything I asked him about and I was really starting to get pissed. I needed some help and dammit, I was going to get it. I tried nice and that got me nowhere. Mind you, I would have been very happy to learn that this was a run-of-the-mill minor foot injury and not something more serious. I needed and wanted this injury to get better quickly so I could go back to work.

I reviewed my symptoms again with the doctor and requested a boot, a referral (to someone who knew what the hell they were doing) and something stronger for pain. The doc repeated his advice for ice, Motrin and rest and turned to leave. I grabbed the back of his lab coat and gave it a little tug. He turned to me with a look of incredulity. I proceeded to tell him in no uncertain terms that I was not leaving without a proper referral, something for pain and a goddamn boot for my foot! He could not get me out of there fast enough...with my boot, a referral and a prescription for Tylenol with codeine.

With x-rays in hand, I saw a podiatrist a few days later. I did, indeed, have a partial tear of the Lis Franc ligament and a small evulsion fracture, which can happen when a ligament is torn away from the bone and the force of tearing breaks off a piece of the bone attached to the ligament. The podiatrist told me that I might need surgery to wire the bones together to keep them in alignment and that I would definitely have severe arthritis in that foot after the injury healed whether or not I needed surgery. *We'll see about that!*

I wound up in a boot for four months and used crutches for minimal weight-bearing. About six weeks in, I tripped yet again because the boot was too big, extending about four inches past the tips of my toes. That little mishap caused a severe sprain in my left ankle, which required wearing a second boot for six weeks. At least now, I had a properly fitting and matching pair of Frankenstein boots for the summer.

At around that same time, I developed severe pain in my right calf. I worried that it might be caused by a blood clot. The podiatrist assured me that it was not a blood clot because I had no swelling, even though I told him that I don't swell much. After several weeks without relief, he decided that it was Achilles tendonitis and injected my Achilles tendon with cortisone, from which I got no relief.

I didn't want to believe that this pain was caused by blood clots so I chose to go along with his Achilles theory. Ultimately the pain subsided, the Lis Franc injury healed nicely (without the need for surgery or getting arthritis) and I went back to work after almost five months…finally.

In retrospect, I can see that I did not bounce back as would have been expected. I had very little stamina and had gained weight from sitting around for those five months consoling myself with comfort food. I seemed to have lost my *joie de vivre*.

Was I depressed? I talked to a shrink who asked me what my first thought in the morning was. Before I even opened my eyes, my first thought was how soon could I go back to bed? I forced myself to stay awake until the street lights came on. When I was a kid, the street lights coming on was our bedtime and I fantasized about shooting them out with my brother's BB gun so I could stay up later. Now I counted the hours until they came back on so I could go to bed. The shrink wanted to know if I thought that the world would be a better place without me in it. *I knew where this was going.* "No, I am not suicidal," I told him. "In fact, I believe that the world is a far better place with me in it." I wanted to drive home my point that I was not suicidal. He wanted to put me on antidepressants. I had taken them years before for situational depression with good results and this seemed like another one of those situations, so I agreed to try them again. I took them for a week and got the raging *squirrelies*. I stopped the meds and saw a therapist, which was a much better choice.

The truth was, I just didn't feel well. Not sick but not well either. Over the next few months, I accommodated this new way of feeling. It didn't really improve. I was having GI (gastrointestinal) issues including cramps, bloating and GERD (gastro-esophageal reflux) and IBS (Irritable Bowel Syndrome). I began to lose some weight without really trying, although I surely wasn't going to complain about that.

In early April of 2009, I had developed the same kind of pain in my left leg that I had in my right leg. I ignored it because I figured it was Achilles tendonitis again, and since the shots didn't help before, I decided to just ride it out. By the end of April, just one year and a day from tripping over that little wee stone, the pain in my left leg had become unbearable. I went to my new primary care doctor, whom I had never met before, and he diagnosed the pain as being caused by a DVT (Deep Vein Thrombosis); that is, a great big blood clot. I argued with him that it was Achilles tendonitis. He was having none of it. At four in the afternoon, just one hour later, I was at the hospital having a Doppler (ultrasound) study done on both legs. The radiologist reported that I had acute DVTs in my left leg and chronic DVTs in my right leg.

Hold on a minute. DVTs? As in more than one? In both legs? It turned out that I had huge clots running from my knees to my groin in the three main veins of both legs. What is the difference between acute and chronic, I wanted to know? Acute means that the clots are still active and are capable of enlarging. Pieces could start breaking off and sail away to far-off parts of my body. The likeliest and most deadly ports of call were my heart, my lungs and my brain. The chronic DVTs in my right leg were well "organized", meaning that they had been sealed over with epithelium, the tissue that lines the inner walls of blood vessels, and posed no immediate danger other than partially blocking optimal blood flow up from my lower leg.

At five o'clock, I was quickly hustled to the Emergency Room to be admitted to the hospital. I needed to be started on blood thinners right away. Intravenous Heparin was the drug of choice to start, as it is fast-acting. They inserted an IV in my left hand and the parade of doctors began. They were the ER docs with their entourage of residents and med students. They called in an infectious disease doctor because

I had this generalized rash that appeared a few months ago and I had been scratching the hell out of it. I had seen a dermatologist – four of them, in fact – and was given hydrocortisone ointment and other lotions that clearly were not working.

Everyone seemed more interested in the rash than the clots. A debate as to whether or not they should give me intravenous antibiotics for a possible cellulitis (a skin infection) ensued. There was great discussion between the ID (Infectious Disease) doc and the ER doc as to whom had jurisdiction to make the decision. After six hours of this nonsense and still no blood thinners, I made the call. I announced that I was not going to be treated with antibiotics since the dermatologist said there was no infection. *My body. My choice.*

It was now eleven p.m. and there was a change of shift. A whole new group of doctors came to see me and review my case. Why has she not gotten antibiotics for the cellulitis yet? *Why the hell have I not gotten Heparin for the f**king clots yet?* I suppose that I should have been frightened by the life-threatening seriousness of my situation, but truthfully, I was just angry. Really, really angry.

Midnight. Eight hours later, I finally got the first dose of Heparin through my IV. It gave me a false sense of protection from the very real threat of a shooting clot with a deadly aim.

Finally, I was admitted to my room around one a.m. I was barely able to sleep with the constant checking of my vital signs and being asked if I was having chest pain, shortness of breath or a headache. *No. Should I?* The concern was that I might shoot an embolism (clot) from my legs to my heart, my lungs or my brain that could kill me. So there I sat all night, terrified and ever-vigilant to the slightest sign of shooting clots.

The question of pain was asked of me by every doctor and every nurse every day for the five days that I was in the hospital. The question was always accompanied by the explanation that I had very severe clots in my legs and a piece could break off and go to my heart, my lungs or my brain and kill me. *I get it, already. I'll let you know. Jeez!*

They started me on Lovenox (a different blood thinner) which is injected into the abdomen. The injections would be discontinued after the dose of the oral blood thinner, Coumadin, was properly adjusted. That was the plan anyway. The wrinkle was that I had a history of a blood clot in my early twenties from birth control pills and was told that I was allergic to Coumadin. Since it was not a huge or very serious blood clot back then, I took baby aspirin for a few months and that was the end of it.

The allergic reaction manifested itself as an itchy rash, hence the dilemma of already having an itchy rash from head to toe of an unknown cause. They would not be able to tell if I was reacting to the Coumadin or whatever was causing the rash in the first place. Dr. Cleary, the hematologist, who ultimately took charge of my case, called in an allergist who doubted that I actually had a true allergy to Coumadin, as it was very rare. The solution was to keep me on the injections twice a day, presumably for the rest of my life because they could not find any underlying cause for the clots. One doctor casually pondered aloud that, finding no other reasonable cause, that I might have cancer. *Cancer! Where did that come from?* She admitted that although I looked way too healthy to have cancer, I should get a Pap smear, a mammogram and a colonoscopy...when I got around to it...just in case.

I was not warming to that idea of the injections, especially since the shots were painful and expensive. Even with my excellent health insurance, my co-pay would have been $2500 per month. There was not even a remote possibility for me to be able to afford that. *What's Plan B?* There was no Plan B. They decided to keep me in the hospital to force the insurance company to relent and pay for the shots. The insurance company responded that I could stay there forever but they weren't paying for the shots or the hospital bill past the five days. The hospital wanted me out because they weren't going to get paid after the five days. *Such a broken system!*

The allergist suggested that they could desensitize me to the Coumadin by giving me a really tiny dose of Coumadin and gradually increasing it. Good idea. I would have to be hospitalized for the process, which would take nine days, but not until the rash that four dermatologists had given up on went away. Each of the four had concluded that it was a stress-induced psychosomatic reaction. The potentially deadly clots and the possibility of having cancer of a yet-to-be determined organ were not really helping my stress level.

On Saturday, the fifth day of my hospitalization, the covering hospitalist (house doctor), who was also the head of discharge planning, was not keen on the idea of keeping me there without the hospital being reimbursed for their hospitality. They couldn't just toss me out without the medicine. *Start thinking outside the box, people!* I suggested it would be cheaper if they gave me a voucher for the injections and I then could be readmitted for the desensitization when the rash was gone. *What a great idea!* They gave me a voucher for a two week supply of Lovenox with instructions not to take the anti-itch medication and to get clearance from *their* dermatologist when the rash cleared up. Great, I had two weeks to get rid of this rash they said was all in my head, when the collective expertise of now more than a dozen doctors had no solution. *There was just no way. I'd had it for months. What magic did they think would happen in two weeks?*

To be clear, this rash did not start out as a rash. I developed what is called an itch-scratch-rash cycle; that is, the itch starts and then you scratch it, which causes the rash. I needed to get rid of the itch in order for the rash to go away. *Tall order.* I am not quite sure how it happened but perhaps through sheer force of will, the itch began to subside to a nearly tolerable level in just a few days while, secretly, I continued to take low doses of the anti-itch meds even though they told me not to take them because they could mask the origin of the itch. Two weeks later, their dermatologist cleared me and I was readmitted to a four-bedded observation unit usually reserved for seriously ill patients as well as for critical care overflow patients for my desensitization process.

Upon admission to the unit, the nurse instructed me to put on a hospital gown and get into bed, as I needed to be hooked up to a heart and blood pressure monitor. Additionally, I would have to use a bedpan since I would not be allowed out of bed to use the bathroom. I informed the nurse that I was not sick and that the first tiny dose of Coumadin would not be administered for another six hours. This apparently was standard protocol for all patients in this unit, usually populated by cardiac patients. I refused and said that I would wait for the doctor to come in. It was not a pleasant exchange.

I understand the efficiency of "standing orders", however, cookie-cutter care does not always apply across the board and I am definitely not a cookie cutter kind of gal. I had made the decision prior to being admitted that I was going to let the authentic, spiritual and metaphysical side of me shine this time. During my first admission, I felt pretty beat up and I had no sense of control over my WellBeing. This time, I was not going to roll over and play dead. I have to admit that I did not win any popularity contests in those nine days and I had to fight tooth and nail to maintain any sense of myself and WellBeing. I was able to get a portable heart monitor so that I could walk in the hall of the main unit. The noise level and negative energy of the other three very sick patients with very upset family members was really stressful.

I noticed that when I was in the unit, I would itch like crazy but when I was in the hall, the itchiness was minimal. I hung out by the elevators during the day and had begun to sleep most of the night in the patient lounge area, although they made me come back to the unit now and then to make a cameo appearance. I passed the desensitization challenge with flying colors and was able to stop the injections and stay on Coumadin. After nine days, I was discharged with instructions to follow up with the hematologist in a few weeks. In the meantime, I would enjoy my medically-mandated summer vacation and try not to worry about the clots and the all-but-forgotten possibility of cancer. *Nothing but clear skies and smooth sailing ahead.*

It turned out that I had little time to sit around and worry about my own situation. My cousin, Ellen, had become very ill with gastrointestinal issues and she was diagnosed with Stage IV stomach cancer in late June. Having the time and being the closest nurse in the family, I offered what advice and encouragement I could. Sadly her disease progressed rapidly and she passed away in late July, barely one month after her initial diagnosis. She was only forty-six years old.

It was sad and scary for me, especially when the words of that hospitalist kept swirling in my head that I might have cancer...somewhere...maybe. But she said I looked too healthy to have cancer. My cousin, Ellen, looked pretty healthy too. I could not even admit to myself that I hadn't really been feeling all that healthy myself.

My follow-up visit with Dr. Cleary, the hematologist, in the second week of August revealed that all appeared to be well. I was tolerating the Coumadin and I had no pain, although my legs fatigued easily with activity due to the impaired circulation. She seemed pleased with my progress and scheduled another appointment in three months. My blood clotting levels could be monitored by my primary care physician. Sounded like a plan to me. As Dr. Cleary was about to walk out of the examination room, she stopped in the doorway, cocked her head to the side and turned around, saying that she was going to order a pelvic MRA/MRV, which is a special MRI (Magnetic Resonance Imaging) of the veins and arteries, ostensibly to see if the clots went higher up past my groin. I saw no reason to be concerned about that, even when she added that I should get it done ASAP. That didn't alarm me in particular either because doctors always want everything done yesterday.

I could have it done on the 16th but that was my birthday. Several years prior, I had a CT scan of my knee on my fiftieth birthday, and it showed that I had a torn meniscus that required surgery. Not wanting to jinx anything this time around, I scheduled it for the 18th and I would see Dr. Cleary the following week. *Back to smooth sailing.*

PART ONE

CHAPTER ONE

THE CALL, THE CHOICE, THE CHALLENGE

The Call
Friday, August 21, 2009

My phone rang just as my client had walked out the door. So much for a breather since the session had run long and my next client was due to arrive in five minutes. Looking at the caller ID on my cell phone, I recognized the number as being from my hematologist, Dr. Cleary, who was managing my care for the blood clots in my legs. I had the special MRI of my pelvis on the 18th and was scheduled to see Dr. Cleary the following week on the 25th to go over the results. I had no concern when I saw her number pop up on the screen. I figured that perhaps her office was calling to reschedule my appointment. It seemed to me that on my last visit, she ordered the test almost as an afterthought. I guessed she was just being thorough and a bit overly cautious. She struck me as a woman who liked to dot her i's and cross her t's.

When I answered the phone, her nurse said the doctor wanted to speak to me. Immediately I could feel the panic rise up in me as if I were being engulfed in flames. That may seem a bit over the top, however, as a nurse, I knew that having the doctor get on the phone in advance of the appointment usually meant one thing – a problem. I croaked out a hello and listened as she told me that the veins in my pelvis were compressed and had impeded the circulation in my legs, which in turn had caused the blood clots to form.

It took me a moment to process that and I asked what was causing the compression. "A mass", she said, "a big one." I went weak in the knees and had to sit down. My head spun. My mouth went as dry as the Sahara. I could not muster a cogent thought. A "mass" is a polite way of saying a big honkin' tumor.

I tried to take a deep breath but I could not. My chest was gripped in a vise of terror and it felt as if only the top half of my lungs could exchange air. Her subsequent questions, which were meant to try and rule *in* some benign possibilities, did little to quell my fear.

I tried to sound reasonable and calm, even though my entire body trembled and I could barely speak above a whisper. The voice in my head, however, was loud and clear. "C'mon, Pat. You're a nurse. You know it's cancer. You're toast." My thoughts went from cancer to fear to pain to death in a nanosecond. I admit that I did not allow for the possibility of anything short of a worst case scenario.

My reaction to the call is known in psychotherapeutic circles as signal anxiety...*on steroids*. Remember that feeling you got as a child when your teacher said, "Put away your books and take out a pen and a piece of paper" as she announced a pop quiz? It was like that, only a gazillion times worse.

I imagine that this call was no picnic for my doctor, either. Since this was not her field of expertise, she asked me if I had a gynecologist and I asked her, "If I see my gynecologist, will she send me to an oncologist anyway?" She said yes, but I already knew that would be her answer. I told her that I would rather just cut to the chase and go straight to a Gynecologist/Oncologist or Gyn/Onc for short. Whatever this thing was, I wanted it OUT OF ME!

The Choice

I soon realized that the paralyzing fear I was feeling was doing just that – paralyzing me from any productive thought or action. I reluctantly and with great apprehension agreed to keep my appointment for the 25th to discuss things more thoroughly.

Blessedly, my next client was 15 minutes late and I took that time to pull myself together. I just had to suck it up and soldier on because that's what nurses do. It never occurred to me to cancel that appointment.

My dear friend and colleague, Lois Brown, joined me for lunch shortly after my last client left and knew immediately that something was not quite right with me even though I thought I was doing a pretty good imitation of business as usual.

A little side note:

The truth is that I am not given to overt displays of emotion even though I feel and experience things deeply. The nuns did a bang up job of teaching us to stuff our feelings. That and nurses were taught to shut down their personal feelings when caring for the sick and dying. Over the years, I did have to learn how to unstuff a lot of emotions and to find a way to express them. But they just don't burst out of me. I joke that if Publisher's Clearing

House showed up at my door with a bunch of helium-filled balloons and a giant check for ten million dollars, my reaction would be disappointingly underwhelming. I would feel great joy and excitement on the inside but what would be captured by the TV cameras would be me quietly accepting the check with a gracious and heartfelt "Thank you, I sure could use this".

To get back to Lois, she is a gifted health coach and practitioner of several CAM (Complementary and Alternative Medicine) modalities which, in broadest terms, means holistic alternatives to traditional medicine. We went to her office and she worked with me using hypnosis and Psych-K (a belief change technique) to push aside the fear long enough to consider that: A.) It might not be cancer, or B.) I could heal myself. Her firm belief from the very first moment upon hearing the news was that I would be fine, indeed, that I was already fine. Lois became the first cheerleader to join my Pep Squad.

It was in those early first moments that I decided I was not ready to die. I was not willing to surrender to the fear. I set about banishing the fear so I could begin to believe that all would be well. *Looking back, I believe that this was a pivotal moment in my wellness journey and I am so grateful that it came so early in my healing adventure.*

It seems ironic that, as a practitioner of several CAM modalities myself, including hypnosis, Psych-K and Emotional Freedom Techniques (to neutralize negative emotions), I told my clients all the time that they were magnificent healing machines and there was no illness too big or too complicated for the body to heal itself. In fact, the client whom I had just seen prior to the call from my doctor wanted to find a way to completely heal her body from Multiple Sclerosis. Our work together included changing her belief system around the inevitable progression of her condition. I sensed that she really wanted to be well with all her heart but in her head, she just could not believe it was possible because logic dictated that the disease would follow a predictably steady course of decline. Now, here I was, needing to put my own belief system to the test.

All this fear and angst and no one but me had uttered the word *cancer*...yet. Of course, being sent to a gynecologist/oncologist because of a huge pelvic mass was a pretty good clue as to what we were dealing with. I knew that, at the very least, surgery loomed large in my very near future. What should I do? Take up yoga? Go vegan? Gluten free? Sugar free? Or all of the above? I knew that there was not enough time to affect any real change in my condition by eating nuts and berries while bending like a pretzel, so I chose instead to create a sphere of WellBeing around me. I chose to focus on healing and wellness. I chose to embrace only positive, life-affirming thoughts and beliefs. I chose to ignore or chase away all negative thoughts and worries. This all sounded good in theory. I didn't know what I was in for, but I was about to find out.

The Challenge

Everything that I had ever learned from my family, from the media, from our society and from my training and experience as a nurse was about to be seriously challenged. I hadn't a clue as to how I was going to do this, yet I knew from the very depth of my soul and with every fiber of my being, that I would find my path back to WellBeing. I didn't know where these thoughts and ideas were coming from. All I knew was that I needed to pull out all the stops and find my way back to WellBeing by healing not just my body but my mind and spirit as well. The big challenge right now was that the surgery would be scheduled very soon and if they found any cancer anywhere, we were talking chemo, radiation and other unpleasantness I didn't even want to think about. Not much time to make it go away or get rid of it, whatever "it" was. I had no plan yet, but my mind was racing to explore the possibilities.

It's been a helluva day and it ain't over yet!

CHAPTER TWO

LET THE HEALING BEGIN

I was still quite rattled when I left my friend, Lois. Feeling the need for a treat, I stopped at a convenience store and bought a bag of those bite-size mini Snickers. I popped a few on my ride home and I began to feel a little better in general. Why Snickers? Not a clue, however, they were to become my go-to treat in the coming days.

When I arrived home, my first call was to my best friend of many years, Pat Evans, also known as The Other Pat, who was at work at the time. She is a nurse and totally unflappable in a crisis. Pat has a background in oncology nursing, so she was a good resource for my many unanswered questions. She also worked at the hospital where THE CANCER CENTER was. *Sounds like a fun place.*

Given her expertise, Pat never showed or expressed any fear for my mortal life as she held on to the hope that it was not cancer. She believed that if it was cancer, in order to be cured, I would still need the whole slash, burn and poison treatment otherwise known as surgery, radiation and chemotherapy. This is gallows humor that we healthcare practitioners sometimes favor to deflect the onslaught of human misery we encounter so often in our daily work.

She was, however, 100 percent supportive of my belief and desire that I could be a part of directing my own healing. *Another cheerleader makes the cut.*

Still needing to talk, I called my friend Sue Nordemo, whom I affectionately call "Snordie". She is also a nurse as well as a Hypnotist and a Reiki Master/Teacher. She was stalwart in her belief that I would be fine and that whatever it was, I would make it all go away. She said I could call and talk anytime, and I did...many, many times. *Cheerleader number three!*

Although I did not know it at the time, this healing would ultimately be accomplished through the integration of traditional allopathic medicine and the holistic healing arts, as well as my rapidly expanding spiritual awakening.

I had decided that until I had more information, I was not going to share any of this news with most of my friends, many of whom were nurses, or my sister, Jean, who was an oncology nurse, because they loved me and would worry about me. I just did not want the energy of their fear and worry about the "C" word to be out there in the ether. It was not that I did not trust that they would be supportive, there was just no sense in everyone getting their panties in a bunch. *In retrospect, perhaps, I should have shared more with them. However, sharing it meant talking about it and talking about it meant thinking about it and thinking about it meant that I was not thinking about healing and that's what I really needed to be doing.*

Where to begin? Good question. I spent the weekend thinking that I could focus on the mass not being cancer but rather it being a benign cyst or growth. A growth is yet another euphemism for a big honkin' tumor. It felt a little like flipping a coin...cancer, not cancer. It occurred to me that this was a 50/50 proposition and I did not like those odds. My new plan was to make whatever it was disappear so that I wouldn't need extensive medical intervention. Good idea but still no plan. I would later learn not to get bogged down in the details of the "how" to do it but rather focus on the "what" to do.

By the following Monday morning, I had decided to call another friend and colleague, Roxy Cortese, whom I had known for several years through our local hypnosis chapter. She is a woman of many skills and talents – massage therapist, Reiki Master/Teacher, reflexologist and hypnotist to name a few. She is, at once, spiritually evolved and yet totally grounded. The truth is that I felt compelled to call her. Not quite sure why at the time but I was soon to find out.

She was able to see me the next day. I told her what was going on and what I wanted to have happen but the fear kept rearing up, seemingly out of nowhere and then I would have to tamp it back down again. It felt like a true contest of wills and it was getting exhausting.

The first thing Roxy did was correct my negative language patterns. I told her of my "problem" and she called it a "challenge". I said I was "afraid" and she called it a "concern". When I said that the facts were undeniably pointing to cancer, she said, "F**k the facts and f**k the cancer too!" *All righty, then.*

Her healing space was dimly lit and soothing new age music with ocean sounds played in the background. The flame of the scented candles flickered, casting shadows on the walls that danced in time to the ocean rhythms. I began to relax immediately.

As I lay on the massage table, Roxy plied an incredibly powerful combination of Reiki and hypnosis that reached into my very core and began to shake loose my negative thoughts, otherwise known as "stinkin' thinkin'". Having been certified as a Master hypnotist for many years and the occasional recipient of Reiki, I was accepting and grateful for her ministrations. She also told me that she was unblocking and balancing my chakras in the process. Even for me, this felt a little "woo-woo", although I felt a calmness that had eluded me in the previous few days. *Soon enough, I would see just how woo-woo things were going to get.*

Wednesday, August 25, 2009

I reluctantly kept my appointment with Dr. Cleary, as promised. I did not want to deal with the reality of any of this. I saw her Fellow first, a young woman from India. She was soft spoken and compassionate and I felt comfortable telling her that I was going to get rid of the tumor. She thought that was a great idea and wished me well. My first declaration to a traditional medical practitioner of my intended self-healing had been well received. I was emboldened to share my intention with Dr. Cleary, who looked at me as if I had suddenly begun to speak in tongues. To her credit, she did not try to dissuade me or correct my wrong-headed thinking. *That went well, I thought.*

Dr. Cleary had given me a choice between two doctors, each having an excellent reputation. I had no personal knowledge of either one, so I let her choose. Dr. Grace had the next available appointment, although she was on vacation for the coming week. *I later discovered that her availability had been another in a series of interventions from the Universe, my Guardian Angel or some other unseen benevolent force.*

No chance to sit idly by. In the intervening days, I was scheduled for a CT scan of my chest, abdomen and pelvis as well as to have blood drawn for a laundry list of tests, some of which were routine and others were, specifically, markers for various cancers. This is all part of what is called a metastatic workup; that is, to see if there is evidence of the cancer having spread elsewhere in the body. And so, the cancer hunt began.

Friday, August 27, 2009

I went for my CT scan. It was a glorious late summer day, the weather was perfect. I would not get the results until I met with Dr. Grace next week, so I decided to enjoy the beautiful day and not think about what the scan might reveal. As I was driving up the road to the radiology center, appreciating a few moments of cancer-free thoughts, my reverie was shattered when I realized that the tree-lined strect festooned with teal ribbons represented Ovarian Cancer Awareness Month and was heralding the unwelcome guest my body currently hosted. There was no escaping the irony. It occurred to me that as I was willingly participating in this cancer hunt, I was also taking my first tentative steps toward unconditional WellBeing.

Still on medical leave because of the blood clots in my legs, I had a lot of free time on my hands to think about my situation and then chase the negative thoughts away. I am blessed with many friends who frequently checked in to see how I was coming along; however, it was difficult to censor my conversations with them. When asked what was new, I would scramble to edit out the trips to the radiology center, the lab for the blood work and the upcoming appointment with the Gyn/Onc.

I was afraid I might blurt out, "I have a gynormous tumor in my pelvis and the doctor thinks it's ovarian cancer. I'm afraid that after being tortured with surgery, chemo and radiation, I will die a slow and painful death. On the other hand, a clot could break off and go to my heart, my lung or my brain and kill me instantly. *Other than that, I'm good. How are you doin'?"*

I was beginning to feel a little lost. I still had no rock solid plan yet so, one evening, I thought I would do something productive or, at the very least, mindless. I decided to clean out my email. I was doing so without paying too much attention. As I was about to push the bulk delete button, one email caught my eye. I didn't know who it was from and it had been sitting in my inbox for at least two weeks. I don't know why I kept it. The subject line seemed innocuous and it didn't peak my interest until that moment. I rarely open an email from someone I don't know, but I had the sense that I should open this particular one.

I opened it to find a link to a ten-minute YouTube video excerpt from *The Science of Miracles: The Quantum Language of Healing, Peace, Feeling, and Belief* by Gregg Braden whom, I later learned, was a pioneer in quantum healing among other metaphysical pursuits. This video snippet showed a woman in a non-medicine clinic in China having a real time ultrasound which revealed a huge inoperable cancerous tumor in her bladder. There were three monks chanting over her. The translation of their chanting was "Already healed". The idea was that they imagined in their mind's eye and in their hearts that she was already well and whole. She was instructed to hold the same thought as well. By some miracle, the ultrasound showed the tumor shrinking and disappearing in just moments, right before my eyes. *Trick photography? A cruel joke? Another sign from the universe? I chose to believe the latter.*

A phrase came to mind that I had heard before but to which I paid little attention. "As the mind goes, so goes the body." I realized that I needed to clean my mental house and keep my thoughts immaculate. Not that I was having impure thoughts that the nuns in grade school assumed we were all obsessed with. No, I just had a lot of "stinkin' thinkin'".

That evening, I must have watched that mystery video at least a dozen times...and many times thereafter. From that moment, my mantra became, "Already healed, I am well".

Hey, it's the start of a plan.

CHAPTER THREE

MEETING DR. GRACE

Wednesday, September 2, 2009

Just two weeks after "the call", I went to meet the Gynecologist/Oncologist, Dr. Grace. I hadn't slept particularly well the night before. *Big surprise!* Despite my positive thoughts and firm conviction that I was well or would be very soon, I was trepidatious. I had never been a fan of being on the receiving end of medical care. I actually have documented White Coat Syndrome; that is, my blood pressure skyrockets when in close proximity to any stethoscope-wielding healthcare professional. I really thought that I would suffer the same level of anxiety as a routine visit to the gynecologist, though I never took into account the fear factor cancer carries with it.

I chose to go by myself. There were people who would have accompanied me, but I didn't want to burden anyone...probably not my best decision. I have always encouraged my clients and patients to take someone with them when going to see a doctor, especially when there was so much at stake. So why did I not follow my own excellent advice? It was not until sometime later that I realized I had some serious issues with unworthiness and undeservedness, but we'll get to that later.

My appointment was for two o'clock and I decided to go early so I could join The Other Pat for lunch at the hospital, which is right across the street from THE CANCER CENTER. *God, I hate that name.* I always got the heebie-jeebies just driving by the place. A little before two p.m., I entered the hallowed halls of THE CANCER CENTER. The lobby looked like a great big bank, cold and uninviting. I found my way to the Women's Gynecological Cancer Suite and presented myself at the front desk. I was greeted warmly by the clerk and given a huge amount of paperwork to fill out. As I sat down in the waiting area, I spied a myriad of pamphlets and magazines on the tables and in the wall racks hawking the wonderful work that THE CANCER CENTER did. Brochures informed me about the early signs of cancer and how it can be prevented. *A bit like closing the barn door after the horses got out, don't you think?* Everywhere I looked...cancercancercancer. *God, I hate that word.*

I filled out the paperwork and chuckled to myself as I realized that in my early twenties, I had very little to report and I would check "no" for just about every disease known to man on the list. At fifty-seven, I had a few more things to check, especially of late. Additionally, when it comes to cancer, they want to know the history of several generations of your entire extended family, living or dead. *Just my luck, I had to come from a very large and very fertile Irish Catholic family. Good thing I had gotten there early.*

Finished, I returned the paperwork to the clerk at the front desk and was handed a folder emblazoned with THE CANCER CENTER name and logo. She told me that I could look through it while I was waiting for the doctor. Inside the folder, I found more information extolling the merits of THE CANCER CENTER and their fine work. There were also stories of cancer survivors and breakthroughs in research. The very last bit was an endowment form in case you wanted to leave your money to THE CANCER CENTER after you croaked. *Let's not get ahead of ourselves, now.* After looking through it, I handed it back to the clerk and told her that I might not have cancer. She told me to keep it anyway...just in case. *Hey, you never know.* I turned to walk back to my seat and as I did, I dropped the entire folder with all of its contents into the wastebasket.

Finally, I was ushered to the inner sanctum and settled in a patient room. It had all the familiar trappings of your typical gynecologist's office: the examination table with the stirrups, the ten thousand watt gooseneck lamp, the rolling stool and the usual assortment of Mengelian-looking surgical stainless steel instruments all neatly arranged on a tray. And, oh yes, more pamphlets about cancer prevention filled a rack on the wall opposite the foot of the exam table. *Not the most pleasant view when peering through your knees with your feet up in stirrups. A Thomas Kincade print depicting a softly lit cabin in the woods, dogs playing poker or an Elvis on black velvet would have been preferable. God, I hate those pamphlets.*

A woman came in and introduced herself as an advanced nurse practitioner, or APN, and without any ice-breaking conversation, she began to pepper me with questions about my health history. *Not getting a warm and fuzzy feeling here.* After about ten minutes, she left the room and I went into the bathroom, undressed as instructed and came out and sat on the examination table with little more than an oversized paper napkin to protect my modesty as I waited...*and waited...and waited for what seemed like forever.*

When the APN came back into the room, she had even more questions. Many of them were repetitious of the ones I had just answered in the reams of forms I had filled out in the waiting room. As if by rote, she went down a list in a rapid-fire staccato, barking one diagnosis after the other in alphabetical order: acne...allergies...anemia...asthma...boils ...botulism...breast cancer...bunions...bursitis and so on. Stopping her several times to give a "yes" response, she would ask for dates. My anxiety was mounting exponentially as time wore on and sometimes the answers didn't come to mind immediately. *Hell, I could barely remember my own name.*

She seemed impatient at my sluggish response time *(my perception)*. I was getting upset. She didn't seem to notice. I was doing my best. I had slipped right back into the good little Catholic schoolgirl mode, trying to get all of the answers right. I was also starting to get a little pissed. I tried not to show it because I didn't want her to get angry with me. She questioned me about cancer screenings and I admitted they were all long overdue. I got a mini-lecture on the importance of keeping up with cancer screenings. *Hello-o-o, barn door.*

Interestingly, the scared, irrational part of me thought that she might be thinking that I deserved to get cancer because I didn't go for the screenings. The rational part of me absolutely knew that this was just not true. *Some crazy stuff goes through your head when you're scared out of your mind.*

When the APN finished her history-taking and a general physical exam, she said the doctor would see me in about fifteen minutes and left the room. No smile. No reassuring word, glance or touch. *All business.* I really tried to make a connection but that shouldn't have been my job. I was scared and suddenly felt very alone.

Soap Box Alert!

Later, in nurse mode, I realized that this nurse was not a villain or acting as judge, jury and executioner. She was overworked and overwhelmed and was, probably, suffering from Compassion Fatigue. This is not an uncommon coping mechanism, especially, among nurses who have depleted their own emotional reserves when caring for patients who are going through cancer treatment. I get that...as a nurse, I totally get that, however, I was the patient and I had enough to deal with on my own. I do not blame her; she was as much a casualty of a very broken healthcare system as I was.

Waiting for Dr. Grace, it, suddenly, hit me that this was for real and if any healing (not a cure) was going to happen, it has to be done by me before surgery or I would be faced with the rather unpleasant options of chemo and radiation. Dr. Grace came in a few minutes later. She was warm and friendly. I gathered the courage to tell Dr. Grace, rather boldly and with more than a bit of false bravado, that I was a practitioner of several alternative healing modalities and that I believed in self-healing and I was going to get rid of whatever *this* was. I further told her that it was important that she accept and respect my beliefs or I was out of there. I was relieved when she simply nodded her head in the affirmative. *I was beginning to feel safe.*

Dr. Grace reviewed the information that the APN had collected and she was very gentle in her approach... conversational, really. She asked me where my family was I told her that they were all over the place: Arizona, Florida and North Carolina.

"No," she said, "who's here with you today?"

"Nobody," I said.

She stopped and just looked at me, incredulous that I came by myself. I told her I chose to come alone because it is my body, my problem and I'll decide who knows what and when. That may seem a little odd to some. Certainly, my doctor thought so.

You see, I was raised to be fiercely independent and to believe that certain things were private. You didn't talk about your salary, your sins or your sex life. I sure as hell wasn't going to bring anybody with me when the whole topic of conversation was going to be about my hoo-ha.

I'm single, have no children and, sadly, I am estranged from two of my three surviving siblings. My sister, Jean, lived in Arizona at the time and was dealing with her own health issues, and I saw no benefit to burden her with any of this since I had no answers at this point. My father had passed and my mother's mind had been whittled away by the ravages of Alzheimer's.

It was time to delve into the family history of cancer. I revealed to Dr. Grace about my cousin, Ellen, who passed away from stomach cancer at the age of 46 just a month prior. I began to cry. She held my hand and patted my shoulder.

Then Dr. Grace went over the results of all the tests. First, she reviewed all those cancer markers that indicate the possibility of cancer in various organs. They were all off the chart and the numbers by themselves meant little to me at the time. She told me not to freak out because there were other things that can elevate the numbers besides cancer, but I wasn't absorbing much of what she was saying at this point anyway. Still, I tried to be helpful by suggesting other possibilities as well. For instance, I was severely anemic, I had IBS, GERD and let's not forget the blood clots. The weird thing was that she said I would need to have a CA125 (a blood test for the ovarian cancer marker) drawn. Odd, I already had it done with the other blood work last week. She suggested that perhaps they hadn't drawn enough blood or the lab forgot to run it. I know that it was done because I made it a point to go over every test on the slip, which included the CA125, with the lab tech because I did not want to have to go back again if they missed something or didn't get enough blood.

At the time, I did not realize how bogus this excuse really was. Much later, I found out that the CA125 was elevated in the extreme from the normal range of 2-34. It was 17,000...that's right, SEVENTEEN THOUSAND! This test was not forgotten or missed. Nobody believed those results the first time around. It is possible to have an elevated CA125 and not have ovarian cancer but let's get real here. There is an old saying that if it walks like a duck and quacks like a duck...it's a duck.

Dr. Grace put the CT scan on the monitor and pointed out a huge blob (*my word for the big honkin' tumor*) about the size of a large cantaloupe around my right ovary and a smaller blob about the size of a lemon on the left side. *Why do they always compare tumors to fruit?* The radiologist's report indicated that the smaller blob was possibly in the uterus or outside of the uterus. Dr. Grace thought the blob was on the other ovary. *Great, a twofer. That really doesn't bode well in terms of prognosis.* She did say that whatever was in there and wherever it was, it all needed to come out.

There was also what is called "ascites" (free fluid) in my pelvis, another ominous sign. The omentum is a fat-like net that gently holds the abdominal organs in place. *Kind of like Spanx for your guts.* Aiding the immune system is but one of the many functions of the omentum. I also learned that if the omentum gets "seeded" with the cancer cells, it can serve as a jump off point for the cancer to spread to other parts of the body. The CT scan revealed shadows that could have been indicative that the cancer had begun to seed the omentum.

A polyp in my stomach was found that looked like a little mushroom. It had a rather formidable stalk or peduncle, like a little tree trunk. I wasn't quite sure what the significance of the thick peduncle was but it seemed noteworthy, at least it was to the radiologist who read the CT scan. A stomach polyp, by itself, is not usually a big deal but when taken as part of the big picture, it may have been significant. Dr. Grace said I would also need to have a colonoscopy and an endoscopy before surgery to examine my esophagus, stomach, small and large intestines for any signs of cancer. There was a possibility that the surgical approach could be very different if the primary site of the cancer was GI (gastrointestinal), meaning that the gynecological issues would take a back seat to the GI stuff and require a GI surgeon to take the lead. Neither option was particularly attractive to me.

Dr. Grace did a thorough gynecological exam and then asked if I had any questions. I asked if she thought I really had cancer. She said she was very "concerned". My interpretation was that I would soon be toast. I asked her if she thought I was going to die and she said we all will someday. I was not feeling very reassured, despite her kindness and gentleness.

I asked for a review of all of the findings. After her recitation, I asked if she had any good news. She looked stumped. I told her I wanted a good news sandwich. This means that the bad news is sandwiched between two pieces of good news. Dr. Grace thought a moment, searching for anything that she could put a positive spin on. The bottom slice of bread was that I was not going to die from stomach cancer. Then she piled on the bad news with extra limburger cheese and onions. The top piece of bread was that I probably did not have cervical cancer. I appreciated that she went along with me and did allow for me to hold on to some hope, although I must admit that the bread on that sandwich was a little thin.

She asked me if I had any more questions. I was too numb to think of any except to ask if she was going to cut through my belly button when she made her incision. Yes, of course. I asked her if she could take a detour and go around it. She said she could do that but I would have a very strange-looking scar. I did not care about that because the idea of cutting through my belly button really skeeved me. I privately thought that this being where I was attached to my mother, it should be kept sacred.

After I changed back into my street clothes, Dr. Grace met me at the nurse's station. She introduced me to the staff and said that in the months to come, we would all become very good friends. *Given my initial introduction, I highly doubted this.* To everyone's astonishment, I asked why we were going to get so chummy. She seemed a bit taken aback and told me that they would take care of me as I recovered from surgery. I accepted that as true. Many months later, I realized that they all assumed that I would be a frequent and unwell visitor as I went through chemo and, possibly, radiation. It truly had not been on my radar screen at this time to even consider that chemo/radiation would be a part of this adventure.

Dr. Grace said she would be in touch as soon as she could schedule the additional testing, the scopes and the insertion of the IVC (Inferior Vena Cava) filter. She called back later that same afternoon. I was to be admitted to the hospital the following Tuesday, September 8. Somehow, I missed the part about being hospitalized for this when I was in her office. Nobody gets admitted for tests anymore. And what about this filter thing? Remember, I had been a baby nurse for my entire career, so this adult stuff was not as familiar to me. The blood thinners had to be stopped so I would not bleed to death during surgery. Stopping the blood thinners would, at the same time, put me at risk to develop blood clots during and after surgery. The IVC filter is a mesh umbrella-like filter inserted into my inferior vena cava (the big vein that carries the blood from the lower extremities up to the heart) to prevent any clots that might develop from travelling to my heart, my lungs or my brain and killing me. *Okay. So it did make sense that if I was going to be probed with semi-flexible tubes up my butt and down my throat that there was a risk of bleeding if they accidently punctured anything.*

And, oh, by the way, I learned that my surgery was scheduled for Wednesday, the 15th of September.

Things were starting to move way too fast.

CHAPTER FOUR

SCOPED, SCANNED, PRICKED, PRODDED AND POKED

Tuesday, September 8, 2009

I was admitted to the hospital to be scoped, scanned, pricked, prodded and poked in preparation for getting sliced and diced next week. Every test and procedure was "diabolically planned" so that I would not be allowed to have any solid food for the next four days. By Wednesday evening, I was so bored out of my mind and starving to death that I actually looked forward to drinking the 128 ounces of Golytely (*what an oxymoron*), a bowel emptying preparation for the colonoscopy on Thursday morning.

The first order of business was to stop the Coumadin, the blood-thinning pill I had been taking for the blood clots. I would need to have Heparin, another blood thinner, administered intravenously. Heparin is a shorter acting anticoagulant and would enter and leave my system more quickly than the Coumadin. This was necessary so that the blood thinners were out of my body for the scheduled invasive tests and procedures and then restarted afterwards. I had to have blood drawn every six hours to monitor the Heparin levels and to adjust the dose appropriately. Other blood work was not coordinated to be drawn at the same time. You see, every specialist had their own agenda so they could have the results when it was convenient for them, which meant getting stuck sometimes every two to three hours. *Feeling a bit like a pin cushion.*

Every nurse and doctor who came into my room kept asking me if I had pain in my legs, pelvis, abdomen, chest or head. Some just assumed that I had pain and asked for a number between zero and ten to rate my pain level. "Nope, no pain," I told them. Why did they all think that I was having pain? *After I recovered from surgery, I realized that I had accommodated and lived with a considerable level of discomfort as this disease insidiously crept up on me over time.*

I found myself with a lot of time on my hands to think about my future...would I have a future? *Cancel that thought.* I would admonish myself for entertaining those negative thoughts that did not serve my highest good and then replace them with better feeling thoughts. More and more the better feeling (high energy) thoughts far outnumbered the negative (low energy) thoughts. If I could not think of an exact opposite thought to counteract the negative ones, I would just think of something more pleasant or watch a YouTube video of a basketful of puppies or kittens or laughing babies...the babies were not necessarily in a basket.

I had not told most of my friends or my sister in Arizona that I was in the hospital. How would I explain my absence? I told my sister I would be away at a wilderness retreat with no cell phone reception. If you met me, you would know how implausible that would be. I made a few brief check-in calls with my friends as I hid in the shower stall of the bathroom so they would not hear the incessant overhead pages.

In between the parade of specialists, Gynecology/Oncology, Hematology, Gastroenterology, Interventional Radiology, Cardiology and a Hospitalist (the big picture overseer), all of whom travelled with an entourage, I focused on my ultimate goal of coming through this odyssey well and whole. This proved to be quite a balancing act, emotionally speaking, when my world of focused healing and wellness collided with the harsh reality of medicine's focus on disease and illness.

Prior to each specialist (an attending physician) seeing me, there were visits from all the members of the entourage: a Fellow (a doctor in advanced specialty training), several residents (wannabe attendings) and medical students (wannabe doctors). Each one would ask the same questions, for which the answers were readily available in my chart. This information was passed up the food chain to the attending physician. Inevitably, this form of communication was about as accurate as playing telephone at a kid's birthday party.

Included in their visits was, for the most part, a cursory physical examination that consisted of a very brief listen to my heart and lungs. I wondered how much information they actually gleaned from this and how valuable it was it in terms of my diagnosis. Now multiply five specialists with four to five members of the entourage plus a nurse on every shift and you get twenty-five to thirty people examining the same damn body part and asking the same damn questions every damn day.

I know that the medical students need some practice with their history taking and their stethoscopic skills, but I had to get on with the business of healing myself. So I finally started refusing to allow some of the underlings to examine me, such as it was, and I even banished one medical student for life.

I wasn't being mean or arbitrary, this guy really pissed me off. I had decided that, while I was not going to interfere with what needed to be done to prepare for the surgery, I did not want to know or be reminded of the ever-mounting evidence for this devastating and life-threatening diagnosis. As a nurse, I knew that many of their findings were ominous and I did not want to focus or worry about the things over which I had no control. I opted, as I said earlier, to keep my thoughts and emotions elevated, as this was something I could control.

The soon-to-be-banished medical student came into my room and began the routine questioning as he flipped through my chart. Suddenly, he began to chuckle. I asked him what was so funny. He responded by saying that he had never seen lab results with such high numbers and began to recite them to me. I told him that I had no desire to know the results, to which he responded that I had a right to know. I told him that I also had a right not to know and again asked him to stop. He just kept reading and laughing. Clearly, he had no concept that these test results he found so amusing were indicators of my possible demise.

Finally, I quietly but firmly told him to leave. He told me he wasn't done yet. *Oh yeah, you're done, pal.* This was our verbatim exchange.

Medical Student: "I have to get this information. What will I tell my resident?"

Me: "You can tell her that you're an asshole, although I suspect she already knows that you're an asshole!"

Medical Student: "You don't understand. I have to finish." He tried to persuade me (begged, really) to allow him to finish.

Me: With great dramatic flair, I said, "Leave this room now and NEVER darken my doorway again! You are banned from my case."

Of course, everything I said after the "never darkening my doorway" part was said to the tails of his lab coat as he beat a hasty retreat from my room. *Sometimes you just have to draw that line in the sand and set some boundaries. It's your body, your life and you are the boss of you.*

Wednesday Evening, September 9, 2009

I was only allowed clear liquids since Monday after dinner and nothing by mouth after I finished the gallon of bowel prep – I had to consume 8 ounces at a time every 15 minutes on Wednesday evening. There I sat, with my chair positioned equidistant between the TV and toilet. *Good times.*

Thursday, September 10, 2009

I was scheduled for the colonoscopy and endoscopy at nine a.m. To quell my nerves, I began to "tap". No, not dance. It is called EFT, or Emotional Freedom Techniques. Generally we just call it "tapping". Briefly, it is thought that all negative emotions are caused by a block in the flow of your Qi (energy or life force). By tapping on various meridian or acupressure points on your hands, chest and face while focusing on an issue and repeating certain phrases, the flow of energy can be restored and release the negative feelings, thoughts, ideas or beliefs. This is a technique that I had been using for many years for myself and my clients with great success. Never before, however, were the stakes so high.

For the next thirty minutes or so I tapped on the various meridian points as I repeated my mantra, "Already healed. I am well" and chanted my healing "Switchwords", which are seemingly unrelated and disjointed words that create a positive effect on the mind and body. I had begun to think of my body as an inhospitable host to an unwelcome guest that gave the cancer no choice but to leave my body. Suddenly, a profound and peaceful calm came over me as if my heart and head were aligned in perfect harmony. My entire being was suffused with a feeling of unconditional love and in that same moment, I heard a voice whisper softly, "You're fine. It's gone". *That's it? No clap of thunder? No heavenly choir? No visit from an Archangel? (Or was there?)* Was it my own wishful thinking or had I just actually heard those words? Yep, I sure did! Despite my momentary doubt and confusion, I knew in that moment my mantra had become my truth. I was already healed and I was indeed well! Just like that, I had the *knowing*.

Moments later, the GI (Gastroenterology) Fellow came to see me. He told me that I would be taken down for the colonoscopy and endoscopy to see what they could find. I corrected him by saying that these procedures were to confirm that all was well. He shook his head in dismay, muttering something about it being the same difference. I just let that one go. I did have awareness that there was a strong suspicion that the gut was, possibly, the primary site or that the cancer had spread there.

I actually felt surprisingly calm. Perhaps a little apprehension but, mostly, I just felt hungry. As the stretcher arrived to take me to the procedure room, the attending gastroenterologist visited me. She was petite and vivacious and each time she said the word "colonoscopy", she would thrust her hip out to the side and point to her butt. She really seemed to enjoy her work!

On the way to the procedure room, I began to feel a little more anxious. I hate having my picture taken and a camera up my butt is probably not my best side. I used some relaxation techniques: self-hypnosis and the tapping. By the time I arrived at the procedure room, I was feeling very relaxed and tired, as I do not sleep very well in those straw-stuffed, plastic-coated mangers that hospitals favor as beds. When the anesthesiologist came in to administer the Propofol (the Michael Jackson sedation of choice), he became very angry and demanded to know who had sedated me. No one had, of course, I was just very relaxed. I understood that it could have been dangerous to administer the sedative for the procedure if I had been given something else without his knowledge. The nurses all denied it, of course, and he asked me if I had self-medicated. I explained that I used self-hypnosis, to which he responded with something between a grunt and a snort. *If anybody needed a chill pill, he did.*

I awakened in what seemed to be the blink of an eye to the sounds of two nurses arguing over who was going to go on a break and who would clean up the procedure room and take me to the recovery room. One of them was shaking my shoulder rather vigorously and shouting for me to wake up. In my stupor, I thought that I was causing the argument and I started to cry while apologizing for making them so mad.

Mini Rant

I tell this story for several reasons. First, the anesthesiologist dissed my beliefs big time. It is important to be respectful of a patient's beliefs and spirituality. Second, when emerging from sedation, a patient's emotions may be rather labile and they are sensitive to loud noises and a non-gentle touch. I found it difficult to assert myself and maintain a degree of dignity when my butt had just been exposed on a sixty-inch plasma screen and as I was still a little stoned. I did not feel that I could be my own best advocate in that moment.

Arriving at the recovery room, I was greeted by a nurse with a sweet smile. I told the nurse that I had cramps and needed to use the bathroom. She told me there was nothing left in there except for the air that was pumped into the bowel to get a better view. She told me that I should just let it out. Much as I enjoy a good fart, I am unaccustomed to ripping them in a crowded room. I realized all the other patients were letting fly and it reminded me of the scene around the campfire in the movie "Blazing Saddles". I was really uncomfortable so I joined in too, although I feared that the gale force wind might cause the stretcher to shoot across the room and hit an innocent bystander.

The GI doc came to see me and told me that everything was perfectly normal. Yippee! I asked her about the stomach polyp and she said, "There was no polyp; just a tiny reddish spot that the biopsy showed to be a slight area of inflammation." Yippee, again. My plan was coming together. Now can I eat? Sure, why not? With that, the radiology doctor came in to tell me that the insertion of the IVC filter that would catch any clots that might form when I was off the blood thinners for surgery had been moved from three p.m. to nine a.m. the following morning. Back to clear liquids until midnight and then nothing...again.

Later, two of Dr. Grace's associates came to visit me in the evening. I told them the good news about the stomach polyp disappearing. *I saw this as tangible proof that the healing had begun since stomach polyps, generally, don't just disappear.* I explained, as I did to Dr. Grace, that my plan was to make it all go away.

They did not share my joy of this little miracle but rather met it with a bit of skepticism. One of the docs offered that the polyp seen on the CT scan was probably not a polyp at all but a piece of undigested food stuck in a fold of my stomach.

Remember the report stated that the polyp had a thick stalk, or peduncle, as we say in medical lingo? *What could have been stuck there?* A peanut was suggested. *A peanut? Seriously?* A whole peanut, pristine and un-chewed attached to my stomach by a thick stalk. That's a new one on me. I am sure they were pulling my leg, as I had never heard of a pedunculated peanut before.

I was undaunted by their unenlightened response. Frankly, that was me not long ago. I was just being authentic and true to whom I had become, which is someone who was already healed and well. I was not going to let anyone's differing beliefs lead me astray from my path. *I'll show them. Just wait and see!*

I was on a roll now and I excitedly shared the disappearance of the stomach polyp with my Pep Squad and received cheers from each one. All of my good thoughts, prayers and intentions to be well, indeed that I was already well, were beginning to pay off. I was so happy that I actually enjoyed my Jell-O, weak tea and greasy beef broth for dinner.

In the evening, after dinner, such as it was, I pondered how much "work" I would have to do to be healed. Have I done enough? Too much? Or was I really to believe that it was truly gone and I was fine? There was really no way to know for sure without another CT scan and that just wasn't going to happen. Pulling out all the stops, I went into hyperdrive, focusing on healing and being well. Later that evening, I achieved a level of deep meditation that has always eluded me, as my mind is rarely still. It felt kind of strange...a good strange.

I was scheduled for early Friday morning for the insertion of the IVC filter. I had previously discussed with Dr. Cleary, the hematologist, that I wanted the filter to be temporary. A permanent filter would have meant that I would need to stay on blood thinners for the rest of my life.

A temporary filter can be left in for around six months before it is considered permanent because the lining of the blood vessel will grow around it. A permanent filter is not designed to be removed at all. Some believed, I am sure, that given the statistical prognosis, it really did not matter one way or the other.

Preparing for sleep and trying to make sense of the enormity of the morning's revelation of the *knowing*, I couldn't help thinking about the procedure I was about to undergo. Having a wire with the filter attached being snaked up through my groin to a point in my inferior vena cava at the level of my upper abdomen was a little scary. Without the blood thinners on board, there was an increased risk that I could "throw a clot".

My father always said that worrying about things that were beyond your control was a waste of time. I chose to embrace that philosophy, as worry is a first cousin to fear and we all know what that will get you.

CHAPTER FIVE

WHO KNEW?

Friday Morning, September 11, 2009

U h-oh! Something was wrong. I awakened to the most incredible, searing pain in my lower abdomen and pelvis. It was like nothing I had ever experienced before. Was this the pain everyone thought I should be having? Did the tumor suddenly explode? Had it leaked and spread everywhere overnight? I was hot. I was burning up but had no fever. I thought that I might spontaneously combust.

Then, I remembered reading about a phenomenon called a healing crisis. It can be experienced in traditional medicine or metaphysically and is also called a spiritual healing crisis. It can cause a temporary or exaggerated worsening of symptoms. Along with the *knowing*, comes the healing. The higher vibration of the healing mobilizes stagnant or dormant energies of the mind and body. Even though this may sound way out there, it actually made sense to me since

I had asked for the healing. I had prayed for the healing. And now I knew for sure that I was receiving the healing.

I hadn't shared my *knowing* with anyone yet, as I was still trying to absorb what the heck happened to me the previous morning. It didn't feel as if what occurred was a revelation of great magnitude or profundity. *Really?* It felt more like confirmation that my intentions were becoming a reality. *Could it really be that simple?* It was one of many miraculous events that I had simply taken in stride, strange as that may seem. Yet they were no less astonishing because having the *knowing* allowed me to accept each subsequent challenge and miracle with seeming ease and aplomb. *Hey, when ya know, ya just know.*

I decided to suck it up and not report the pain to the nurses or doctors. When asked, I just smiled and said I had no pain. Why should I incite a whole new round of tests and speculations? Ignoring the pain, I felt an optimistic anticipation of what was before me. All was right with the world. *My world, at least, and that's all that really mattered to me.*

As a general rule, I do not recommend anyone to keep that kind of information from their doctor. I felt confident in my knowing that it was all part of the healing crisis.

The Filter

I had been preparing myself mentally and emotionally for several days prior to the insertion of the IVC filter. There were so many ways this procedure could go awry. Even with the *knowing* that all was well, I spent my time before the procedure "tapping" away the anxiety that was threatening to overwhelm me. It was not long before I realized that I was no longer afraid about the procedure itself. The only fear that remained was that I would have to use the bedpan if my bladder couldn't wait the six hours I was required to stay very still and lie completely flat after the insertion of the filter so that the puncture in my groin would not start to bleed. A lab tech came to take a blood sample to determine my blood type in case I needed a blood transfusion during the procedure. I jokingly told her that I didn't need the test because I already knew my blood type. It is the same as my philosophy of life...B-Positive. She very seriously explained that she still had to take the specimen. Perhaps she thought that if I got angry, my blood type might change to B-Negative.

It was time to go for the filter insertion. Arriving at the interventional radiology department, my stretcher was parallel parked in a hallway with a dozen or so other patient-occupied stretchers. The interventional radiologist (IR) came to speak with me and to have me sign the consent for the procedure. I read it carefully to make sure that it specified a temporary filter, which it did not. I modified and initialed that omission and shared with the doctor that my hematologist, Dr. Cleary, had requested a temporary filter to be inserted. He seemed annoyed when I asked him to check her original request. I could not figure out why that should make any difference to him.

In the procedure room, a nurse came to clean the skin at the insertion site. Imagine my surprise when he asked me to turn my head to the left and placed a surgical drape over my face. I asked why he was prepping that area. The nurse told me that the filter would be inserted through my neck. *Whoa, hold on there, cowboy.* There was never any discussion about the neck. All prior discussion about the filter was that it would be inserted through the groin. I asked to speak to the IR before I would allow the nurse to continue the prep. Annoyed once again, the doctor said that in looking at the CT scan, the size of the tumor would make passing the filter through the groin impossible. *Okay, that's reasonable, however, not a big fan of those kinds of surprises. The possibility of using the neck was never mentioned and I had a right to know, even if I had no objections.*

As casually as *oh by the way*, the doctor then informed me that he was going to insert a <u>permanent</u> filter through my neck. Now, get this. The reason was because they did not have a <u>temporary</u> through-the-neck filter in stock! I told the doctor that this was unacceptable, to which he responded that I had no choice. Did he really want to go there? *You just don't ever want to get a redhead's Irish up!* I could feel my blood type changing from B-Positive to B-Negative.

Thank goodness I had not been sedated because I really needed to stand up for myself, which was not an easy task being naked under a sheet, flat on my back with both arms strapped down. I mustered up as much indignation and outrage as I could under the circumstances and told the doctor that in no uncertain terms would I make a permanent and life-altering decision because the filter was out of stock. I did not care which way it went in as long as it was temporary.

Not wanting to screw up his schedule or cause the surgery to be postponed, the radiologist opted to do an ultrasound of the groin area for a better point of view and to see if it might be possible to insert the filter there. What occurred next was another one of those little miracles that were becoming a regular occurrence. After viewing the ultrasound, he said that the tumor appeared to be smaller than the CT scan and the MRI had shown it to be originally and he thought he would be able to go through the groin after all. *My, my, my...how about that!*

The procedure went flawlessly, although my anxiety level skyrocketed. I don't believe that I was given any sedation. If I had been sedated, it was not enough. When the time comes to take this sucker out, I want to be snowed.

Back in my room, I tried to nap, but it just wasn't happening. I was hungry and thirsty and I had to pee. Damn, it's only been four hours and I still have two to go. Finally I had to bite the bullet and ask for a bedpan. This may seem like TMI but the flat, tiny fracture pan used for patients who must remain flat in bed is mounted by rolling to your side as the pan is jammed under your butt and all this while trying not to put any strain on your abdominal muscles. Reversing the process would be even dicier and with my vast experience as the giver of bedpans, I knew this all too well. Removing a fracture pan brimming with fresh hot steaming urine without a major spill requires very steady hand. Let's just say that I was treated to a bed bath and clean sheets for my efforts.

Finally, I was able to relax and I decided to watch TV. There is always an episode of NCIS with my man, Gibbs, on some channel at any given time. I was getting pretty bored and my back was aching from being flat all day.

The Consent

Late in the afternoon, Dr. Grace came to see me. Even though it was Friday and my surgery wasn't scheduled until the following Tuesday, she wanted to discuss the surgical options, possible scenarios and to have me sign the surgical consent. I felt comfortable that we would have an open and honest exchange. We chatted a bit, just girl talk, and then she eased into her pre-surgical shtick. Dr. Grace was very thorough in her explanations and did not make assumptions that just because I was a nurse, I knew what the heck she was talking about. Most of my career was spent taking care of babies, not where they came from.

I was surprised by the myriad of options she explained that covered every possibility depending on where and how far the cancer had spread. I really thought she planned to just gut my pelvis by removing all of the reproductive organs and the tumors. She went into great detail about rearranging muscles and ligaments in the pelvis or possibly re-plumbing my bladder or rerouting intestines and explaining the repercussions or physical limitations that might occur as a result.

Dr. Grace was very animated in her presentation and for some reason, I found this all to be rather amusing and I began to chuckle. She asked me if I understood everything and if I had any questions. I asked her how long this would take. Six to nine hours. I told her that I didn't want her to have to work so hard and that all she needed to do was remove the unnecessary parts and offending bits.

She looked at me quizzically and asked if I had taken a tranquilizer, knowing that she had not ordered any. For the second time in two days, I was asked if I was self-medicating. I replied that I had not and she wanted to know if I was on antidepressants. Nope, not them either. Apparently, I had been grinning like a Cheshire cat. Perhaps out of frustration or exasperation, she placed her arms akimbo and said, "You have no fear, no anxiety. Where does this come from?" I told her that I had a *knowing* that all was well and that when she opened me up, she would find things to be very different than she was expecting. She wanted to know how I knew. *Hmm.* It is difficult to explain a *knowing* to someone who has never experienced a *knowing*. You just know when you have a *knowing*. Truthfully, I did not know what a *knowing* was until I had my own *knowing* and then I just knew.

I did think about it a bit and finally told her, "When you look at me, you see a woman riddled with cancer, but when I look in the mirror, I see a healthy vibrant woman and that is who I want you to operate on!" I had naively thought that she had taken my word for it when I said that I was going to heal myself.

I signed the consent and as she left, I am sure she must have considered a psychiatric consult, as I was clearly in denial if not delusional. The truth is, Dr. Grace never wavered in her support and respect for my beliefs and philosophy.

The plan was to discharge me the next morning and I would be readmitted early the next Tuesday morning, the day of surgery. I was anxious to go home. I had plans for a massage in the afternoon and a big steak dinner with friends in the evening. I had to content myself with pot roast smothered in congealed gravy and cold instant mashed potatoes for the evening meal. *At least it wasn't clear liquids.*

Shortly after Dr. Grace left, a very bright young Gyn/Onc associate, whom I affectionately thought of as Baby Doc, came to see me. I was a little surprised by her visit but any friendly face was welcome. She told me that my Pap smear results came back as grossly abnormal and highly suspicious of cancer. I would need to have a colposcopy (a microscopic inspection of the cervix) before surgery. I questioned the need for this procedure since the cervix would be removed along with everything else. Baby Doc explained that the cancer may have spread differently than they originally thought, so depending on what was found, the surgical approach may have to be changed.

She seemed really upset and was apologetic about being the bearer of more bad news. I just laughed and told her not to worry because that Pap smear was two weeks old and I was sure my cervix was already fine. *As I heard myself talking, I wondered who had commandeered my mouth.*

Baby Doc appeared to be relieved by my reaction to this new wrinkle and said she liked my positive attitude. It was so much more than a positive attitude, but I didn't have the wherewithal to go through the whole *knowing* thing again. I told her before she left that I needed to be discharged very early in the morning as I had much to do. It hit me that I would be laid up for some time after surgery and needed to get my ducks in a row in addition to the massage and the steak dinner. She assured me that she would be in bright and early in the morning.

The pain was still there but I somehow was able to ignore it, confident that it was all part of the healing process. Despite the pain, I was able to fall asleep easily and slept like a baby that night.

A Weekend Pass

Saturday, September 12, 2009

As promised, Baby Doc came to see me at about eight a.m. and said that she would start the discharge process. The paperwork required for discharge has gone beyond ridiculous. There is far less paperwork if you croak. At one p.m., I was officially discharged and went directly to see Roxy for my massage. I was still wearing my PJs, as I had no time to go home and change.

I had an incredible massage with Reiki and more Chakra balancing. After the session, Roxy and I chatted awhile. I was relaxed and we had some laughs and gossiped a bit. As I was getting ready to leave, Roxy showed me a drawing she had done on a yellow legal pad. It depicted the reproductive system, loosely speaking, with "OK" written over the right and left ovaries and a small dark spot on the uterus with the words "not to worry". *I'll take it!*

Before I left, she gave me some healing Reiki in my hands that I was to give to Dr. Grace right before the surgery was to begin. I did not quite understand this but I was game for anything.

Dinner with friends was a nice distraction, though still a challenge to edit my conversation. I was also wearing long sleeves on a very warm night to hide the bruises left from the

IVs and needle sticks. *I guess I could have told them that I had taken up self-flagellation.*

Sunday was spent cleaning and doing laundry and making lists. I'm big on lists. I make checklists for everything. My mother would have been so proud. She loved lists. Only thing is, I would usually lose them before I could actually check anything off. I watched some TV, ate a few bite size Snickers and went to bed. It was still rather strange for me to feel so completely at peace and I slept really well.

Monday, September 14, 2009

No chance for sleeping in, I returned as promised at seven-thirty a.m. to THE CANCER CENTER for the colposcopy. I guessed I would have plenty of time for sleep after surgery. *Yeah, right?* By eight a.m., the exam was over and my cervix was found to be in pristine condition; no sign of cancer, infection or any other abnormality. *Damn, I'm getting good at this!*

CHAPTER SIX

SLICED AND DICED

Tuesday Morning, September 15, 2009

The day of surgery had finally arrived and I was due to report to the admitting department of THE CANCER HOSPITAL at ten o'clock a.m. I was facing an uncertain future and this day would determine, to some extent, what that future might be; yet I was still feeling pretty confident in the *knowing. Is this what faith is?*

I went through the usual paperwork dance, answering the same questions and providing the same information as I had done countless times in the previous several weeks. My best friend, Pat Evans, met me in the admitting area and we made our way to the surgical waiting room. Along the way, I had to stop to use the restroom. When we arrived at the surgical waiting room, I realized that I had left one of my many forms in the bathroom. *Can't get in without the golden ticket.* Pat handed me the rest of the papers to hold on to while she retrieved the missing form. *I was still feeling pretty calm and relaxed but I wish someone could have told my bladder that.* As I waited outside the pre-op area for Pat to return, I glanced at the top sheet of my bundle of papers and saw the copy of my Operating Room schedule that lists the patient's name, time of surgery, assigned OR room, the diagnosis and the procedure to be performed.

And there it was, right there on that little half sheet of paper:

Name: Crilly, Patricia
Time: 2:00 pm
Room: 2
Diagnosis: Invasive Ovarian Cancer
Procedure: 1. TAH/BSO (total hysterectomy and removal of both ovaries and fallopian tubes)
2. Metastatic Staging (getting a definitive answer as to the extent of the cancer)

And that's when I lost it. My head swirled. My stomach heaved. I felt dizzy. Dr. Grace didn't believe me! Had she just been humoring me all this time? She must have thought it was going to be really bad. I did all this work for nothing. *So much for the knowing. So much for faith. I'm going to die!*

With that, Pat returned to find me decompensating in the hallway. Not outwardly, of course. To the casual observer, I was just another patient waiting to be called in for surgery. The only tell was the uncontrollable trembling of my hands as I showed Pat the paper. Unflappable as always, she explained (as the rational me already knew) that it is standard procedure to stage the cancer regardless of the doctor's personal beliefs, feelings or hope for their patient. Pat said that it would be perfectly acceptable for Dr. Grace to go in and find nothing. She reminded me that I had to have faith in my *knowing*...that I was already healed. That simple reminder and her steady presence was enough to get me out of that tailspin. It was just that I had never associated cancer and me in the same sphere. *Whew! That was gnarly.*

Back in my Zen-like state again, I was ushered into the pre-surgical area, where I was given a "Johnny" coat (a patient gown) and directed to my little cubby, replete with hospital green curtains and a stretcher with an IV pole. Dr. Grace came in and said everything was ready and that the surgery would begin on time. Good, because once again, I had only clear liquids all day and had to do the Golytely bowel prep...again...and then nothing after midnight. At least I would not feel hungry while under anesthesia.

I asked her if I could listen to my iPod in the OR. I had made a recording that began with the song *Ordinary Miracles* performed by my friend and favorite singer, Maureen McGovern, followed by healing affirmations that I had recorded for myself. Dr. Grace said no one had ever made that request before but it was fine with her. We needed to check with the anesthesiologist first because the iPod would be in his work area.

The anesthesiology Fellow, who had come to do the pre-op check and start my IV, said that she would speak to the attending anesthesiologist about my musical request. I also told her to tell him that I had a history of being extremely combative and really cranky when coming out of anesthesia.

After about fifteen minutes, which seemed like a lifetime, the Fellow returned to report that the anesthesiologist was not comfortable with me having my iPod in the OR. The reason was that he did not want to take responsibility for it if it got lost, broken or stolen. *Oh, come on!* This was really important to me because if I croaked during surgery, I wanted the last thing I heard on this earth to be the voice of an angel and not the cacophony of shouts, alarms and worried words. I offered to sign a waiver absolving the hospital and its employees from any and all responsibility for any loss, theft or damage to my iPod. He finally agreed, with some reluctance. *Seriously? This was 2009. Patients were bringing in boom boxes with cassette tapes and 8-tracks back in the '70s.*

In the meantime, Ari, a medical student (no, not the asshole), came in. That's when I found out that he was going to start the IV. Remember, I had spent the last week as a human pin cushion, so finding a big fat vein was going to be slim pickin's. I learned after the fact that this was his first attempt at starting an IV, which was a recipe for disaster. I told him he got one shot at it. He failed...miserably. He also dropped the needle on the sheet between my knees. That is a big no-no because people tend to forget to pick them up or they get lost in the bedding and someone could get stuck, preferably not me. Pat's sharp eye caught his faux pas and disposed of the needle appropriately. The Fellow got the IV in easily. *Good thing because she was only getting one shot too, or I was going to put it in myself.*

Pat wished me well and promised to be there in the recovery room when I woke up. Since I had no family here, I had given my permission for Dr. Grace to talk to her and share any information necessary. In fact, I signed for Pat to be my medical proxy, giving her the right to make all medical decisions for me if I became incapacitated. Right on time, they wheeled me into the OR. I scooted onto the OR table. *Damn, it was cold!* They quickly covered me with warm blankets and I put my ear buds in. The circulating nurse said she would hit the start button on my iPod before they knocked me out. The anesthesiologist took two wide foot-long strips of adhesive tape and secured my iPod with an "X" across the left side of my chest. *That's gonna smart when that tape comes off.* For good measure, he stuck three or four hospital issue labels with my name, birthdate, room number and religion on the iPod itself.

Dr. Grace came into the OR before she did her scrub to assure me that she would take good care of me. Of this, I had no doubt. Remember that Reiki energy Roxy had given me?

I asked Dr. Grace to give me her hands and I held them in mine for several moments. Her hands were strong but soft and I could feel her compassion flowing through them and into mine. It was very comforting. I told her that my friend had given me Reiki energy to put into her hands so that the moment her scalpel touched my skin, I would begin to heal. She thanked me and left the room. When I looked around, everyone was standing still and staring at me. *Jeez, I was just being true to myself. I guess these people didn't get out much.* I turned to the anesthesiologist and told him that I could go to sleep now. The circulating nurse pressed play on my iPod and listening to the dulcet tones of Maureen McGovern, I slipped into the arms of Morpheus.

Some time after ten o'clock p.m., I awakened with a start in the recovery room (now called the Post Anesthesia Care Unit or PACU). I had difficulty focusing, especially without my eyeglasses. There were a lot of voices and a lot of activity. Then I saw Pat and I tried to sit up but I could not. My hands were tied down. I kept asking, "Am I alright?" but no sound was coming out. I felt the panic rising up in me. The nurse told me to relax. She said that everything was all right but the endotracheal (breathing) tube was still in my throat. I tried to pull the tube out but of course, my hands were restrained. I felt a combination of panic and anger. I wanted that tube out. I wanted to speak...to be heard...to ask if I was okay. My words were unheard, however, I believe that I got my point across. Pat tried to calm me down but I would have none of it. As if out of nowhere, Dr. Grace appeared. She had actually been there all along but I guess my field of vision was somewhat narrowed from the effects of anesthesia and sedation. She told me that the tube was in because I had gotten too much anesthesia and I didn't wake up in the OR. *Well, I'm awake now!* "Do you want the tube out, Pat?" *Duh? Ye-ah.* She instructed the nurse to have the anesthesiologist come and take out the tube. Why do we need him? That could take forever. *Let me take this f**king tube out myself! I'm a nurse, goddammit! I know how to do it.* When the tube was out, I could finally ask if I was okay. Dr. Grace said that the tumor was a low-grade cancer and everything else looked clean so far. She told me that I would still need a little chemo. *A little chemo is like being a little bit pregnant.* She asked if I would agree to that. *Sure, why not?* Even in my haze, I *knew* that the final pathology report would be clean. Besides, I had no strength to argue at that point.

I was drifting in and out, as they had given me another dose of morphine, probably just to shut me up. Apparently, in addition to being combative, I was also quite chatty once the tube came out. As they were preparing to transport me to my room, I heard Dr. Grace shouting. Well it sounded that way but everything was sounding kind of loud. She said no one was going anywhere until my iPod was found. *Oh, no! It's the hospital's worst nightmare come true. I bet they're sorry that I didn't sign a waiver.* The empty iPod case was there, still taped to my chest. After a frenzied search, my iPod was found stuck in the guts of the underbelly of the bed. It must have slipped out of its case during my struggle to break free of my restraints.

Finally around midnight, I arrived at my room. They very carefully positioned and locked the stretcher next to my bed. As four people gathered to transfer me from the stretcher to the bed, I heard the words that I had uttered many times before, never appreciating the gut-wrenching pain that would ensue for the patient. "Bend your knees and scoot your bottom over a little bit." *Sweet Lord in Heaven! That is a pain that's gonna linger. Break out that morphine stash.*

Finally, I was tucked in and ready to try and ignore the searing pain. I just wanted to go into a state of oblivion by sleep or drugs. I didn't really care which. The rest of the night was a series of catnaps punctuated by nurses and techs coming in to draw blood, take vital signs and fuss with the IVs. I had been told that I would have a "pain pump" that would deliver continuous pain medicine via the IV. It was not helping.

Wednesday Morning, September 16, 2009

At five-thirty a.m., Ari, my medical student, appeared to examine me. "Can you sit up?" *No.* "Can you *roll* over on your side?" *No.* "I need to listen to your lungs." *You figure it out, I'm not moving.*

Around seven a.m., the covering surgeon, who was not Dr. Grace, came to visit with her crew and wanted me to sit up or roll to my side. *Still not gonna happen.* She removed the bandage to check my incision, revealing a ten-inch line of staples, resembling a train track from just above my pubic bone, up my abdomen with a slight detour around my belly button and back to the midline for another inch or so. The surgeon said it looked beautiful. *In the eye of the beholder.* She left the incision open to air. I asked if I could shower and she said perhaps in a day or so when I felt up to it.

When asked about my pain level, I told her that I had terrible pain all night without any relief from the medication. She looked at my chart and said that what was ordered should have been enough to help with the pain. The nurse was asked to check the pump to see how much medication was given during the night. "None" was the answer. *What? None!* Apparently, the pump was not set for automatic pilot with a "rescue" dose that is patient controlled at specific intervals. Why didn't I press the button myself when I had pain? *Didn't know I had a button.* I don't recall having that pointed out to me but I was not at the top of my game the night before. *Oh, wait. There it was draped over the headboard far out of my sight and reach.*

Mini Rant:

That is just basic patient care 101 to make sure that the patient has the call button and pain control button within easy reach. It is usually tethered to the side rail.

The night nurse had reported that I never asked for anything for pain during the night. I was unable to muster the strength even to speak. I think those little catnaps were actually me passing out from the pain. The doctor remedied that situation with apologies and really ramped up the dosage. *Yes! Thank you.*

I had cotton mouth and bed head and I wanted to take a shower. No bedside birdbath for me. Pat arrived before her shift began and helped me into the bathroom, dragging along the IV pole with several pumps attached to it along with my urine bag. This was against her better judgment but the doctor said I could *(kind of)*. She knew that there was no point in arguing with me.

By the time I reached the bathroom and arranged my toiletries, I was overwhelmed with fatigue and pain. As the spirit may have been willing, I had to reluctantly admit that the flesh was indeed too weak for a shower. I grudgingly opted for the birdbath. I blew my hair dry and put on some lipstick and blush. It's not that I am such a girly-girl; I was afraid that my fair skin and natural pallor enhanced by the anemia might have the doctors thinking I was in worse shape than I already was.

Pat helped me on with my jammies, which consisted of a long-sleeve cotton tee shirt and cozy fleece sleep pants. This was no simple task. The IV tubing had to be clamped off and the tubing disconnected so I could get my arm with the IV into the sleeve. The tubing connected to the catheter in my bladder had to be snaked down the leg of my jammie bottoms. Thirty minutes later and I was feeling human again. I was tired and hurting...bad. *Time to push my rescue button.*

I chose to sit in an upholstered chair instead of getting back into bed. It was a shorter trip and easier to get into. Pat and I sat for a few minutes before she had to officially start her work day. The hematology Fellow came into the room and looked at me and then at the chart and back out into the hall to check the room number again. He said he was looking for Patricia Crilly. *Yup, that's me.* He said, "No, the patient I'm looking for had major surgery late yesterday afternoon." I told him that I was, indeed, Patricia Crilly. He thought that we were visitors and trying to play a joke on him. As proof that I was the patient for whom he was looking, I held up my right arm with the IV and my hospital bracelet. *Amazing what some snappy jammies and a little blush and lipstick can do for you.*

I got back into bed and Pat left for work. I was exhausted. Baby Doc came in a little while later and marveled at how well I looked and said that later on the nurse was going to help me get out of bed to sit in the chair for fifteen minutes and I was not to give her a hard time, explaining that I needed to start moving and walking. I told her that I had already been up, bathed and had sat in the chair...twice. She told me I was doing too much and I did not have to prove anything by showing off. I protested. I was not showing off. *Well, okay, maybe a little.* I had no problem with sitting in the chair. It did hurt to sit in the chair but it hurt just as much sitting in the bed.

In the afternoon as I lay in bed trying to find just the right spot to ease the pain even a little bit, I realized that it was September 16th, my mother's eighty-fifth birthday. *Happy Birthday, Ma.* I felt a pang of sadness that she could not be here with me. With her advanced Alzheimer's, she could not even muster a cogent thought to wish me well and blessedly, nor could she fret or worry about me. The essence of the mother I loved and who loved me had long since gone. She always had a will of steel and her body stubbornly refused to let go. I had a fleeting thought that if she would just surrender instead of languishing in a state of limbo between this world and the next, she could be with Jim-Boy (my dad) and watch over me from heaven.

Dr. Grace finally came by to see me. Noticing that the dressing had been removed, she asked me with a rather self-satisfied smile on her face if I noticed that she had made the incision around my belly button instead of through it as I had requested. I told her that I did see that and jokingly told her that I wanted her to go around to right of my belly button instead of to the left. I don't remember much of what we talked about but it was comforting to have her there. I felt that when someone cuts you open and digs around inside you, shoving their hands all the way up under your diaphragm, a special bond is forged for life.

During the late evening, the nurses were in and out hanging IV mini bags and fussing with the IV pumps. It seemed a little excessive to me. I asked what was going on and I was told that my kidneys were not making urine, so they were giving me what they called a fluid challenge to kick-start my kidneys. I should have been alarmed by that but I had enough painkillers on board not to worry. Sometime in the wee hours of the morning, I felt like my bladder was going to explode. I really felt like I had to go. Impossible, said the nurses, because I had a catheter in my bladder and any urine in there would drain out into the bag. I felt that if I could stand up, my bladder would empty. This was not rational, obviously, as girls do not have to stand up to urinate. With all the surgical activity in that area, it was hard to tell what was going on down there.

Thursday Morning, September 17, 2009

In the morning, a nephrologist came to see me and explained that because of the extra anesthesia, my blood pressure had bottomed out during surgery and put my kidneys in shock. *OMG! I was in kidney failure!*

I went into nurse mode to think rationally about what this meant in terms of my healing which only made me catastrophize about all of the possible ramifications. How would I manage chemo (if I needed it) and kidney dialysis at the same time? I felt the fear that I had so assiduously kept in abeyance begin to creep in again. *Wait a minute. I had the knowing! Would the angels have whispered in my ear that the cancer was gone just to have me die from kidney failure? Nope. No way. I contented myself that, with the promise of this miracle, the urine too shall come to pass.*

On the heels of that less-than-stellar news, I was informed via email by my estranged elder sister that my mother had a stroke and was not expected to survive very much longer. I was flooded with conflicting emotions. Had my prayers been answered? Was it the selfish prayer that I wanted her to watch over me? Was it the loving prayer that wished for her to find peace? It was a little bit of both, I think. Honey, as everyone called my mother, was stubborn, indeed, but her timing was impeccable. Some would say it was a coincidence. I don't believe in coincidences. It has been said that a coincidence is God's way of remaining anonymous.

I spoke with my sister, Jean, asking her to intervene on my behalf as I did not want to learn of my mother's passing via email. Jean called my other sister and told her that I was in the hospital recovering from surgery for ovarian cancer and not to contact me when Honey passed. I had maxed out on the allotted pain medication and it did little to quell my emotional pain. Now I just had to wait for the other shoe to drop...two shoes, actually. I could only sit and wait to hear about my mother, and I had to wait to hear about the final pathology report because my prognosis was still officially up in the air. *This was not one of my better days.*

CHAPTER SEVEN

PAIN, PAIN GO AWAY

Friday, September 18, 2009

Like clockwork, at five-thirty a.m., my medical student, Ari, awakened me by tweaking my big toe. *Do they teach them that in med school? It's really annoying.* Can you sit up? *No!* Can you turn to your side? *Maybe.* I managed a quarter turn to my right side. He asked me to turn a little more. *Man, you give 'em an inch!* I told him not to push his luck. I was feeling a little snarky.

Afterwards, the surgeon (no, not Dr. Grace) came in to check up on me and changed my pain meds from IV to PO (by mouth). I was still having a lot of pain. With an injured limb, you can isolate that part when looking for a comfortable position. When it is your abdomen, any movement for any reason triggers the pain right to the very core of your being.

Pain is now considered the fifth vital sign right up there with pulse, respiration, blood pressure and temperature.

This makes sense because pain can throw off your other vital signs for a negative impact. It is routine to ask a patient what their pain level is between zero (no pain) and ten (worst pain ever). Mine was hovering between an eight and a nine despite the medication. The pain meds were only taking the edge off. On admission, I was asked by the nurse what was an acceptable level of pain for me. I said zero. That would be unrealistic, I was told. I insisted that zero was my acceptable level of pain even though it was doubtful that this could be achieved. Pain perception is subjective, after all.

A little side note:

When I was in my early twenties, I had to have my wisdom teeth removed. This, I was told, would be very painful. Not being a fan of pain, I read about alternative means to ease pain and came across an article that said moaning was very good for pain relief. It said something about the vibration of the moan matching the vibration of the pain. Worth a try. A few days before the procedure, sitting in my parents' house, I started to moan...very loudly. My mother asked what I was doing and I told her I was practicing.

After the wisdom teeth came out, I went home and lay on the couch and moaned...loudly. Everyone went into the kitchen and I followed them and continued to moan...louder. Jean told me that they accepted that moaning could be therapeutic but did I really need an audience? In my somewhat addled pain medication-induced state, I said yes. I explained that it is like the age-old question about a tree falling in the forest and if no one is there to hear it, does it really make a sound? I am that tree in the forest, I told her. If there is no one there to hear my moans, do I really have pain? It made sense to me at the time.

I have long been the butt of jokes from family and friends that I am a major weenie when it comes to pain. It always made me feel weak and inadequate. I learned years ago that it is what it is and I do not need to tough it out to show that I can take it.

I do not believe in stretching out the time between doses until the pain is unbearable. Consistent blood levels of pain medication make it easier to manage the pain without the highs and lows. I didn't mind that it made me groggy and foggy. I had nothing to do and nowhere to go. I had no fear that I would become addicted as I had no desire to be in an altered state when mental alertness was required. *I JUST DON'T LIKE PAIN!*

After a couple of days and still taking the pain meds every four hours, a nurse commented that she could set her watch by my request for pain medication. *Is that a bad thing?* The pain was real and yet I felt, once again, that I was showing weakness. *And then I thought, f**k it! You switch places with me and they'll be setting the US Naval Observatory Master Clock by you!*

I was thinking that it was time to venture forth into the hallway and take a little stroll. Up until then, I had been just walking around my room and to the kitchen for ice chips. Walking was good for me to do. Any movement was good after surgery, especially walking. It helps the circulation and wakes up the intestines. I grabbed my IV pole with the two pumps attached and my urine bag and peeked my head out of the door. There were about a half dozen women leaning on their IV poles and dragging their urine bags as they slowly shuffled up and down the hallway. They were young and old, many were gray and ashen. Some wore the mask of death I had seen too many times before. My gut wrenched to see their suffering.

I stepped out into the hall and I modeled the other patients' gait. I hunched over, leaned on the IV pole, put on a mask of pain and slowly shuffled one circuit of the unit. As I rounded the corner near the elevator, I was greeted by a very fancy and very large sign welcoming one and all to the Women's Gynecology Cancer Unit. As the elevator doors opened, I was met with a few pitying smiles from its occupants. How pathetic I must appear. Bent over and shuffling made me feel weak and vulnerable. I made another circuit of the unit only this time I stood up straighter, which happily did not cause additional discomfort, put a smile on my face and pulled my IV pole along with me. What a difference in my sense of WellBeing.

I retreated back into my room and took a good look at myself in the mirror. I truly did see a healthy, vibrant woman. It was at that moment that I realized the magnitude of what was happening to me and the blessings I was receiving.

I was looking forward to the afternoon. My friend, Lois, and her husband, Chris, were coming for a visit. My first visitors other than Pat. I had not felt up to it before. I went to take a shower and noticed that my legs had ballooned to about twice the size of normal. The sight was quite alarming; although my normal is not exactly Twiggy-esque, my legs looked enormous. They looked like tree trunks and I even had "cankles"! The fabric of my sleep pants was stretched tight across my thighs. I realized they felt heavy and a little achy. It felt as if I was walking through a waist-high snow drift.

The nephrologist said that it was part of the kidney failure, however, I was beginning to make a little bit of urine. Well, that's good news, but what about the swelling? I could barely get my little scuffy slippers on my feet. She told me that this would diminish over the next three or four weeks. No, this needed to go away sooner than that. I will put that on my list of things that need to be healed ASAP.

Time for lunch. Finally, after nearly two weeks of clear liquids and almost no solid food, I was allowed to have a regular (anything on the menu without restrictions) diet. It is true what they say about no longer feeling hunger after food has been severely restricted, however, I was starting to feel hungry and eagerly awaited the arrival of my lunch tray despite it being hospital food. My tray was finally delivered and much to my disappointment, I had no appetite!

Lois and Chris visited for about two hours and we played a game called Rummikub. I don't have any recollection of actually playing the game but apparently, I won! It was good to be with friends and just talk about stuff, the kind of stuff that has nothing to do with urine production, blood work and such.

In the evening, I spoke with a few friends on the phone and each expression of sadness about Honey's stroke and the trips down memory lane made me weepy. It seemed strange to me that none of the nurses offered any comfort or support to me regarding my diagnosis and presumed prognosis, yet they were all solicitous about my mother's imminent passing. The nurses were all nice to me and responsive to my physical needs, however, not one of them ever touched me except when necessary to perform a task and always with gloves on. I get the whole universal precautions thing, but I was beginning to feel like a leper.

Soapbox Alert!

Now, I know things have changed since I worked in a hospital back in the Stone Age and sadly, not for the better as far as I can see. Nurses have a lot more responsibilities these days, which has taken them further and further away from the bedside. I am not indicting my nurses or any nurses for that matter. I do call out the nursing profession, in general, for what it has become. Nurses have gone beyond being paper pushers to being techno geeks where much of the patient interaction occurs with a computer between the nurse and the patient as she/he enters the data into a rolling computer station.

I need to talk about the olden days when I was a young nurse, which I swore I would never do when I got to be an old nurse, but here goes. I held my patients' bare naked hand in my bare naked hand. I hugged them and their family members. I cried with them in their sorrow and celebrated their joy. We talked about their physical, emotional and spiritual WellBeing. I got to know who they were.

I worked the evening shift early in my career on a men's medical/surgical floor. I was twenty years old when I started. Part of our routine was to render PM care. Today that means Post Mortem care. Back then it meant evening care when we "tucked" our patents in for the night. We straightened their sheets or changed them if needed. We filled their water pitcher, helped them wash their hands and face and brush their teeth. We gave each and every patient a two or three minute back rub which, as my freshman nursing instructor, Mrs. Edith Sistek, taught us, includes the buttocks because that's what they were sitting on 24/7. We were able to assess our patients from head to toe while we offered support and comfort.

PM care was not an option if time permitted. It was as sacrosanct as giving the patient their medications, changing their dressings and taking their vital signs. This is a practice that has gone by the wayside along with love beads and hip huggers. Nurses just don't have the time for it anymore and that makes me sad. Okay. Off my soapbox...for now.

As I went to sleep for the night, in between the vital sign checks, IV medication and blood draws, I wondered why I had not seen Dr. Grace. I felt abandoned. I was beginning to think that she had, as we said when I was a kid, "left me flat". I really thought we had bonded. Maybe tomorrow. *Hopefully.*

Saturday, September 19, 2009

Talk about setting your watch. Ari, the med student showed up at five-thirty a.m. sharp. This time I was ready for him. I had learned a new trick during the night. I was able to turn all the way over onto my right side, my preferred sleeping position. I had also tucked my feet up so there would be no tweaking of my toes. You'd think he'd be impressed. No, he asked me to turn over onto my left side. *Really?* I did not feel the need to impress him but an "atta girl" would have been nice. I felt he must be punished for his transgression so I would not let him look at my incision line. I needed a little bit of control in my life and his assessment was for his benefit, not mine. *Still feeling a little snarky and perhaps even a bit peckish.*

The covering surgeon came in after having had a discussion with the hematologist. They were putting me back on Heparin (the IV blood thinner) which had been held back because of the kidney failure. I did not realize that I had not been getting it. It was more important than ever to get out of bed and keep walking so I wouldn't get any more blood clots. She asked, as she and every other nurse and doctor have been asking every day since surgery, if I had moved my bowels. Apparently, I had no bowel sounds when they listened to my abdomen with a stethoscope. Things get sluggish after anesthesia, taking pain pills and being relatively inactive. It can cause a great deal of difficulty in getting the choo-choo to leave the station. *The thing they failed to understand was that there was no choo-choo in the station!*

I asked her why I had not seen Dr. Grace, and she said that it was not her week to cover the surgical patients. I was told not to worry because they kept her apprised of my progress. It felt like a bait and switch to me. I felt sad. *Where is the continuity of care? Where is the personal attention? We bonded, dammit!*

The nephrologist came in the early afternoon and announced that my urinary output was greatly improved. *Yippee! Can you take out the catheter, because I really feel like I need to pee?* Okay, but if you do not produce sufficient amounts of urine, we will put the catheter back in...*over my dead body!* I was able to go shortly after the catheter was removed which, by the way, had gotten inadvertently kinked sometime during the night and was not allowing my now-filling bladder to empty completely. I had to go every hour or so, but I was passing greater quantities each time. Each drop was measured so there could be no cheating.

She scheduled an ultrasound of my kidneys for later in the afternoon. *An outing, how fun.* In addition to the kidney failure thing, a very large stone had been discovered in my left kidney on the original CT scan. She told me they needed to make sure all was well with my kidneys before the chemo started. I told her that I had not discussed that with Dr. Grace and that chemo may not be necessary.

"Oh, you're having chemo," she said.

"I will see what Dr. Grace has to say," I replied.

"No, you *are* having chemo!"

I thought to myself, just let it go. *You're not gonna get the last word in with her.* I knew this discussion would come, but I honestly did not see myself having chemo. When I thought of the future beyond this adventure, I would be tiptoeing through the tulips happy and healthy.

I was taken to radiology for the ultrasound in the very late afternoon. I had to bend my knees and "scoot" onto the table...without any assistance this time. The table was hard and cold and there were no warm blankets coming as they had in the operating room. An ultrasound requires turning in a variety of positions to get a 360-degree view as they move a lubricated wand over your abdomen. I was slow to move and the technician was impatient, rough and, quite frankly, nasty. *I had a few suggestions as to what she could do with her ultrasound wand.*

As I tucked myself in for the night, I felt a little bit at odds. I had hoped to be discharged three or four days after my surgery. I have now completed post-op day three, and there has been absolutely no discussion about sending me home. *Nurses don't make patient patients.*

CHAPTER EIGHT

THERE'S SOME GOOD NEWS AND SOME BAD NEWS

Saturday, September 19, 2009

The Good News

The good news was that I was moving around a lot better. I was turning side-to-side in bed and getting in and out of bed without feeling like I would, literally, spill my guts. I was practically doing wind sprints around the unit every hour or so. Okay, maybe not wind sprints, but it felt like it. Interesting that one of the nurses asked me, "Where's the fire?" and admonished me to slow down. I was frequently cautioned to take it easy because I was doing too much. *Are you kidding?* I was the ideal patient. Most patients have to be prodded and scolded and at times badgered to get out of bed and walk.

It is also a good thing to cough and breathe deeply to make sure your lungs are expanding and so that mucous doesn't settle in your chest, which would increase your risk of getting pneumonia. A few days earlier, just clearing my throat would produce an exquisite level of pain. After surgery, each patient is given an incentive spirometer which is a clear plastic cylinder with a ping pong ball inside and a piece of corrugated plastic tubing about an inch in diameter attached to the bottom. The idea is to suck in on the corrugated tube with all of your might to make the ball move up the cylinder, sort of like making the bell ring by swinging the sledge hammer on the Strength-o-Meter in an amusement park. It was painful and I did not find this activity particularly amusing. At about three a.m., as I lay awake, I realized that I had not been coughing nearly enough. I began to cough for several minutes with as much vigor as I could muster. The night nurse came in with a look of distress and asked if I was all right. *Yes, I'm fine.* Why are you coughing so much? *No particular reason. Just thought it was a good idea as long as I was up.*

I was doing everything I was supposed to and they kept telling me to slow down. I wasn't showing off anymore. My recovery was remarkably swift, as was attested by each doctor and nurse who cared for me. "Amazing" was a word I was becoming accustomed to hearing. What I didn't realize at the time was just how sick I was supposed to have been.

Speaking of sick, I told my friends not to send me any flowers because they remind me of a funeral home and no get well cards either because I am already well and never really considered myself to be sick. In honoring my request but wanting to show their support, a bouquet of helium-filled Mylar balloons was delivered to my room. Some had big smiley faces and others just said "Congratulations". They made me happy each time I looked at them.

A little side note:

I awakened later in the wee hours of the next morning and saw movement at the foot of my bed. All I could make out in the dark was some type of creature about four feet tall with an oddly shaped head that seemed to be dancing back and forth, never taking its eyes off me. It made no sound. Was I dreaming? Could this have been an alien abduction? I was a little frightened. I switched on the light and to my relief, I realized that one of the smiley-face balloons deflated slightly and had broken away from the pack and gone rogue. Time to lay off the drugs.

Pat came to visit later in the morning and brought silicone bracelets I had made up when my cousin Ellen was so ill. They were teal and embossed with purple lettering that said, "**I Believe in Miracles!**"

I had encouraged Ellen's family to continue to hope and pray for a miracle but the news got worse with each passing day for my cousin. Sadly, the bracelets arrived the day of Ellen's funeral. Little did I know at the time that I would be the one to be the recipient of not just one, but many miracles.

I chose the color teal because it is the color of healing. It is also interesting to note that it is the color for Ovarian Cancer Awareness Month, which I did not know at the time. *Coincidence?* I decided that I would give them to the staff, nurses, doctors, housekeeping, dietary and anybody who came in contact with me. I left them in a little basket on my nightstand and invited one and all to help themselves. I was gratified that everyone seemed genuinely touched and began wearing them every day. It gave me an opportunity to talk about my healing with the staff. One lady from dietary cried when I gave it to her because she had a sick adult child who needed a miracle. Many people shared their own stories of healing and faith and miracles.

A lovely woman from housekeeping came in and asked if she could have another bracelet because she knew when her daughter saw it, she would snatch it right off her wrist. She came in several days later without her bracelet and sheepishly admitted that she had given hers to her pastor at church. I gave her several more. Others began to ask for another bracelet to give to a friend or family member.

Up until that time, I had felt rather invisible. Finally, I began to have some meaningful exchanges with the staff and felt for the first time that they were seeing me as a real person.

Mini Soap Box Alert:

The nurses' assignments were constantly being adjusted to accommodate the flux in the patient census. If someone went home, the nurse was assigned another patient. If a nurse got an admission, one of her patients was reassigned. Even though the nurses worked twelve-hour shifts, I was frequently assigned to a different nurse every four hours and rarely had the same nurse twice. How can nurses get to know their patients as anything more than a diagnosis and a room number? Very sad. Heartbreaking, really.

The rest of the day was spent just hanging out and visiting with Pat and a few friends who stopped by.

Sunday, September 20, 2009

The Bad News

I awakened on my own quite early. Who can sleep with the constant nocturnal visitations from nurses, lab techs and med students? I actually enjoyed my breakfast for the first time in quite a while. I was looking forward to another visit from my friends, Lois and Chris, later on.

I took my shower later in the morning. I was feeling a little lazy. As I stood in the shower, I heard what sounded like a high-pitched gust of wind barreling through the bathroom. Just as suddenly, I saw or thought I saw an emerald green mist quickly blow past me and disappear into the shower wall. It was a little disorienting. Perhaps it was the pain medication. Then just as suddenly, I knew – yes, it was a *knowing* that my mother had passed.

I stood in the shower and wept until the hot water went cold. Even though I had long since said goodbye to Honey, I was stunned at the depth of my sorrow and yet rejoiced to know that she was finally free of her corporeal prison. My sister, Jean, called shortly after to tell me that Honey was gone. Not surprisingly, it was at the exact time I had the *visitation* in the shower. I could confirm the time because I am never without a watch, even in the shower.

Each nurse and doctor that came in always asked about my mother, and today was no different except that telling them brought another wave of grief and tears. One of the residents (I can't remember which medical specialty) was the first to ask about Mom on this day. My tears flowed and I could barely speak between the sobs. Words weren't really necessary, but apparently the resident thought they were. She sat next to me and wrapped her arms around me and began to rock me. It was comforting. Then she started to scream, "Stop your tears! Your mother is dead! She doesn't matter anymore! You must put your energy into getting well! You were a good daughter and you must focus on getting well. That is all that matters!" There was a bit of a cultural divide here about death and dying, but I appreciated her attempt at comforting me nonetheless.

To throw a little more fuel on my sadness, I started thinking that I was not always a good daughter. Sometimes I really sucked at being a daughter. In her earlier stages of Alzheimer's, I got to know a whole other side of my mother and she saw another side of me. Her driving need for perfection was the first to go. We came to have an appreciation of each other and while others lamented her downward spiral, I cherished that time with her.

I remember as a child when one of my classmates lost her mother. I thought, how can one go on? How could you ever speak of her without tears? I was never comfortable crying in public. How would I ever get through the funeral if I lost my mother?

But we Irish are a stoic lot. It was always a point of great admiration for others and a source of pride for my mother when one was strong and held up well in the face of the death of a loved one. I held it together when my friends called to offer condolences; that is until the Eucharistic Minister came to visit. I am no longer a practicing Catholic, although I got plenty of practice through twelve years of parochial school and three years in a Catholic nursing school. Even though I consider myself to be a recovering Catholic, my personal concept of God remains an ever-present constant in my life.

I refused communion and the minister offered a blessing. I accepted the blessing but told the minister that I felt I was underserving of it since I was not the best daughter I could have been and should have been. She told me we are all flawed human beings and that my mother and God had already forgiven me. More tears. More sobbing. I really needed to suck it up. Crying gives me such a headache. *I maxed out on the pain meds. Grief is exhausting.*

Monday, September 21, 2009

More Good News

The doctor who had insisted that I would be having chemo came in and told me that the final pathology report showed that the tumor was borderline...not normal but not cancer. She told me that I would not need to have chemo after all. *I told you so!* I was thrilled, of course, though not surprised by this news and it was a relief to finally have confirmation. I might have even danced a little jig had I not been in so much pain both physically and emotionally. *But why, I wondered, didn't this news come from Dr. Grace?* The doctor sharing this news then added without skipping a beat that while it was not cancer now, it could come back again as cancer. *Gee, thanks for giving me thirty seconds to enjoy my miracle.*

There were those over time who speculated that I never had cancer in the first place or that it was a spontaneous remission. There was nothing spontaneous about this healing. I WORKED MY ASS OFF! One would think that, working on a women's gynecology cancer floor, this kind of news, which is rare indeed, would be cause for rejoicing, for celebration with high-fives all around. *Nope. Nothing. Nada. Nyet. Not even a blip on their radar.* I found that to be perplexing and sad.

My visit with Lois and Chris gave me some respite from my sadness and we were able to enjoy the good news that I had done it. I set out to be healed and it came to be. I can't help but think that my mother found a way to intervene on my behalf.

I was exhausted from the roller coaster of emotions. I hoped that I would be able to get a much-needed restful sleep, as I was already having some serious sleep deprivation what with the blood work, vital signs and IV medications all through the night. *I just wanted to go home.*

CHAPTER NINE

IT'S COMPLICATED

Monday, September 21, 2009

Okay. I have had it! I have got to get some uninterrupted sleep. The unit nursing supervisor came to check in each day, and each day she said that I was sent her very best nurse. *More like five or six of her best nurses every day.* She always asked if there was anything I needed. *Yes, a good night's sleep.* I told her that I decided that I was not to be disturbed between midnight and six in the morning. No blood work, no vital signs (as long as I was stable...which I was), no meds, no med students, no nuthin'. She told me I would need the doctor to order that. *My body, my decision. I was not going to take no for an answer.*

The surgical gang came early to make their rounds. I told the surgeon of my plan. She asked if the nurses could make their rounds through the night. *Yes, but no shining a flashlight in my face or talking to me. The only reason to disturb me was if I was dead.* We were in agreement. Later in the day, my nurse put a sign on my door which read, "**Do NOT Disturb from 12 AM to 6 AM per patient request.**" Ari, the medical student, asked if that meant him as well. I told him anyone who entered did so under threat of death.

A discussion ensued among the surgeon, Fellow and residents as to whether or not they should remove the staples from my incision. What did I think? I did not have strong feelings one way or the other. I was more interested in what Dr. Grace thought. Well, you know they say she is a little conservative. Dr. Grace had not seen the incision, so I went with their decision. *You snooze, you lose, Dr. G.* Besides, there was a possibility that I could go home the next day...if I moved my bowels. *These people were bowel obsessed.* The surgical resident returned a little later and took out the staples...all thirty-six of them. They were beginning to pinch a little so I was glad to have them out. After my shower, I sat on the side of my bed and felt a *pop* and then a *rip.* I looked down to see a wet stain spreading across the front of my sleep pants. Well, at least it wasn't blood because I really didn't have any to spare. I rang for the nurse who looked at my incision, slapped a combine (a surgical dressing that looks a bit like a sanitary napkin) on it and fetched the resident back.

The bottom two inches of my ten inch incision had split open. I felt a burning sensation. Not to worry, it happens a lot, I was told. So I had to have what is called a wet-to-dry dressing applied to the wound. That means they soaked a 4x4-inch gauze pad with saline (sterile salt water) and placed it over the gaping wound and then applied a combine over it, taping it securely to my abdomen. I was assured that this would not delay my discharge the next day. The tape was pulling at my skin and was way more uncomfortable than the pinching and itching of the staples.

The rest of the day was spent quietly. I felt a little numb, not really able to feel the depth of my grief and not able to feel the joy of my restored WellBeing. I tried to look forward to going home in the morning...if I pooped. At least the thought of going home helped to take my mind off the loss of my mother for brief periods.

Later in the afternoon, Dr. Grace made an appearance... finally. She asked if I had heard the good news and I nodded yes. She told me that the pathologist called to say that she had made a mistake. The tumor was not cancer. *I can live with that kind of mistake.* It really was not a mistake. The specimens that are examined during the surgery do not yield as detailed an analysis of the pathology as the in-depth analysis that takes several days to examine all of the tissue thoroughly.

Without going into a lot of medical detail, all of the areas that looked "suspicious" were biopsied and upon initial inspection during the surgery, they looked like cancer. The final pathology report revealed that the twenty or so biopsies of suspicious-looking tissues taken from lymph nodes, my omentum, my diaphragm and the outside of my bowel were all areas of inflammation, not cancer. *Hmmm, interesting.*

There was necrosis (dead tissue) in the center of the tumor, meaning that it had begun to die from the inside out. This usually occurs with chemo when the blood supply to the cancer is disrupted. Surprisingly, the uterus, which looked grossly normal, had a very low-grade, non-invasive cancer for which the cure was the hysterectomy. Was not expecting that but it was all good. I forgot to ask about the second tumor. Clearly it was gone when they got in there since there was never any mention of it in the operative report or the pathology report. I am guessing that the little bit of cancer found in the uterus had once been that lemon-sized second tumor.

Dr. Grace said that I was right and she was wrong. No, we were both right. The cancer was there and then it went away as I said it would. I thought of it as a recession of the cancer rather than a remission and the areas of inflammation were just the remnants of the cancer that had once been there. I often thought that had I waited another week or two, it all would have been gone. The nurse in me would not allow me to wait and that was okay. I was happy with the results.

Dr. Grace asked about my mother. I just shook my head and said she was gone. She hugged me...tight. Then I hugged her...tight, and I thanked her for believing in me. Then I scolded her for not coming to see me every day. She explained that it was their system of rotating duties through surgery, clinic and hospital rounds and I told her that their system sucked. I felt buoyed by Dr. Grace's visit nonetheless and felt that everything was working out as it should.

I had been eating solid food for several days and figured that there must have been something to move along by then. I was just one little poop away from going home. *I wondered if farting counted.* It was difficult to tell if the twinges I was feeling in my abdomen were an urge to go, the gaping incision or the residual surgical pain. After dinner, I decided to go into the bathroom and help Mother Nature and the Dulcolax (stool softener) along.

I apologize in advance for the graphic description about a bodily function that is generally not discussed in polite company, however, it is an integral part of my journey.

While on the commode, I strained a bit to see if that might get the ball rolling, so to speak. It was painful to stress my abdominal muscles as they had been surgically split right down the middle. I also worried that I might further dehisce (tear open) my wound.

After a few minutes, I felt that success was at hand, when suddenly, I heard what sounded like a gush of urine hitting the water, only it did not feel like it was coming from my bladder. On closer inspection, I realized that it was coming from my rectum. I had, in layman's terms, "popped a hemorrhoid", and it was bleeding profusely. I was embarrassed and tried to clean up. My attempts only made things worse. I pulled the emergency call button, alerting someone in the nurse's station that there was an emergency in the bathroom.

First the nurse's aide arrived, and with a look of shock and horror, she announced that she would get the nurse. A moment later, the nurse showed up. The blood was still flowing like an open spigot. I was hemorrhaging...profusely. The two of them helped me to a chair padded with towels and blankets. I explained to the nurse what had happened and she said she would be right back to help me get cleaned up. Looking back into the bathroom was reminiscent of a scene right out of *CSI*. I guessed that I wouldn't be going home in the morning.

Forty-five minutes had passed and no one had come back. I was not near a call light and I was afraid to stand up. I was feeling pretty woozy and lightheaded. I did not know if I was still actively bleeding. My door had been closed over so no one could hear my cry for help. I got up from the chair and travelled the three or four steps to the bathroom to reactivate the emergency switch. I was relieved to see that the bleeding had subsided. The aide came in and I asked if she could help me get cleaned up. I kept apologizing for making such a mess. She was very reassuring and kind.

The nurse finally returned with apologies for the delay saying there was an emergency with another patient. *It must have been a humdinger to trump a hemorrhage.* Back in bed, the thought came to me that it was the blood thinners that had caused the excessive bleeding when I strained even moderately. I should have known better.

I mentioned previously that I was already in a significant state of anemia. This little stunt must have really put me over the edge. Whether or not anyone ever came back to check on me is hazy. I know that I was emotionally, mentally and physically compromised. Patients in crisis do not make their own best advocate.

Tuesday, September 22, 2009

It was three a.m. and I had been sleeping soundly when I was awakened by a lab tech who flipped on the overhead light and none too gently dropped his blood-drawing basket on my bed. I looked him square in the eye and told him that if I wasn't dead, he had better get his butt out of there. A nurse appeared and told him he was in the wrong room. He beat a hasty retreat.

I was feeling pretty whipped when I was awakened by Ari at six a.m. on the dot. I was shaky and weak when I went to take my shower. I caught a glimpse of my face in the mirror and was horrified at how pale and drawn I looked. There was not enough blush and lipstick in the world to mask my Casperesque appearance. After my shower, I did not take a walk. I did not sit in the chair. I got right back into bed. I lay there feeling that my mind, body and spirit had been under siege.

During the surgeon's visit during rounds, I was told that my hemoglobin had dropped significantly. *Big surprise!* I was asked if I would agree to a blood transfusion. It's not that blood transfusions are like playing Russian roulette because of AIDS anymore, but they are given more judiciously now. Still, it gave me pause. I agreed to it as I knew it would take months to build my iron stores back up to par, and I was already compromised by the anemia. I was weak. My heart rate was elevated and I was short of breath with minimal exertion. I needed the transfusion.

I had a unit of blood infused in the afternoon, quickly followed by a second unit. I was feeling like I had a little more pep by the evening.

Wednesday, September 23, 2009

I was actually able to sleep through the entire night, from midnight to six a.m. anyway. Six hours of uninterrupted sleep was just what the doctor ordered...*at my insistence, of course.* Feeling almost human again and relaxing in the chair, I looked back over the previous evening's events and several things stood out for me as being pretty scary in terms of my safety and WellBeing. I had been left unattended while actively bleeding. The aide should have been instructed to stay with me while the nurse called the surgical resident STAT! No one ever checked to ascertain exactly where the bleeding was coming from. They took my word for it as to its origin. Had this been vaginal bleeding, it could have been a true surgical emergency. No one checked my blood pressure or checked my blood count during this event. I know that my blood pressure was checked at some point later on. How much later, I had no clue. I chose not to dwell on this and just be grateful for my many recent blessings.

When the surgeon and company arrived, I was happy to report that the choo-choo had finally left the station. She was happy to report that my hemoglobin had increased significantly after the two units of blood the day before and I was cleared to go home. *Going home. Music to my ears.*

The hematologist came by shortly after the surgical gang had left, and I asked when the IVC filter could come out since I no longer had cancer which can contribute to the formation of blood clots. She suggested that we wait a few weeks until I was more fully recovered. I had been through enough. *Fine with me.* As she turned to leave, she stopped, cocked her head to the side, turned back to me and said that we might as well have it removed before I went home and just get it over with. I could go home later in the afternoon. *Fine with me.*

I was taken to the Interventional Radiology Unit and was met by a very gregarious and kind radiologist, Dr. Rand, who was to do the procedure. He was as different as could be from the guy who put in the filter. Dr. Rand had a reputation for being among the best of the best Interventional Radiologists. I told him that I did not want to be awake for this procedure as I had been the first time. *Fine with him.* Just as Dr. Grace had, he reassured me that he would take good care of me.

The filter must be removed opposite the direction of its insertion, so my head and neck were draped and I was given Propofol and off to La-La Land I went. Sometime later, the drape was lifted and Dr. Rand bent close to me and said, "Hello". I asked if he was done already. Propofol makes time feel like it passes in a nanosecond. No, he said he couldn't take the filter out. *Why?* Because there was a great big free-floating clot stuck on top of the filter. *Well, suck it out!* Can't, it doesn't work that way. *What are you going to do?* I'm going to put another filter in through your neck to trap it. *Why didn't you just do it instead of waking me up?* It is a different procedure and I need your permission to do it. *Fine with me but just make sure it is a temporary filter!* You're going back to sleep now. As he was drawing the drape back over my head I heard him say, "Good thing they sent her down today or she would have been dead." Then boom! Back to oblivion.

Something I didn't ponder until later was that just attempting the removal of the first filter, there was a possibility that the clot could have been dislodged and shot to my heart, my lungs or my brain and killed me instantly. Putting another filter on top could have dislodged the clot and killed me instantly. So if Dr. Rand hadn't awakened me with the news of the clot and it did kill me, the last words I heard would have been of comfort and reassurance from him. So being awakened with the news of the new clot, the last words I heard would have been a harbinger of my impending death. Not a comforting thought.

I further thought that if the hematologist had not changed her mind about waiting to take the filter out, I would have croaked at some point for sure. I don't think Honey had any idea just how busy her first week in Heaven was going to be. *Thanks, Ma.*

The hematologist came back as I was in the middle of my six hours of lying very still with my head elevated precisely at thirty degrees. She acknowledged the close call and said that I could go home as planned in a few hours. I had come perilously close to death twice in two days. *I'm not going anywhere.* Although in retrospect, home might have been the safer alternative. These last two incidents really scared the crap out of me. Even though the hematologist felt it was safe for me to go home, she agreed to keep me one more night. *Good thing, 'cause I wasn't goin' nowhere, no way, no how.*

Thursday, September 24, 2009

Finally, I was going home. I had been hospitalized for fifteen out of the last eighteen days. It had been quite a ride. As I waited for my friend, Donna, to take me home, a most unexpected thing happened. A nurse by the name of Kaye, who had been assigned to me on my first surgical admission on September 8th, stopped into see me. I had seen her on the unit and hoped she would be my nurse every day. She was always assigned to the most difficult cases. She would wave and say hello when she passed my room. Today, even though she was not my nurse, she said that the unit was very busy but that she had some time and would make sure I had everything I needed to go home.

For the better part of an hour, she gathered my dressing supplies, my prescriptions and got me a red rubber donut for my tender butt as well as an abdominal binder to hold the dressing in place because the tape had begun to tear up my skin into a bloody pulp. Kaye went over everything, even though, as a nurse, I knew this stuff. She hugged me and expressed her joy at the outcome of the surgery and my good prognosis. She held my hand and offered me words of encouragement.

Kaye is the embodiment of what a nurse is. Her level of caring and expertise was extraordinary and yet it is the minimum we as patients are entitled to. Thank you, Kaye. Thank you to all of the nurses who toil each day in a broken system that does not support you in your desire and ability to render the care your patients so desperately need and deserve.

I'm outta here!

CHAPTER TEN

HOME SWEET HOME

Friday, September 25, 2009

So happy to have slept in my own bed. A little bit strange too. It took me about two hours for my morning rituals, as they had to be adjusted to compensate for my snail-like pace and to incorporate the packing and dressing change of my open wound. I made my way slowly downstairs. Each step was a little jarring, as my "going downstairs muscles" were way out of practice.

What to do? I didn't have to do anything and yet I could do anything I wanted, taking into consideration my physical limitations at the time, of course. I felt a bit like a fish out of water. I wondered if this was how it felt to get out of prison and be able to choose freely without monitoring or restriction. This may sound a bit melodramatic, however, everything had changed. Even though I was okay, life was different. I was different. I was physically, emotionally and spiritually different. Not necessarily in a good or bad way…just different. Okay, mostly in a good way. It was going to take time to adjust to my new way of being.

After breakfast, which turned out to be an early lunch by the time I got downstairs, I was ready for a nap. The Other Pat was ever vigilant that I not overdo. Don't think I could if I tried. Several weeks earlier, I had made an appointment with Doris Cruz for the afternoon, thinking I would have long since been home and well on the road to recovery. She is a compassionate, intuitive and spiritually-gifted therapist whom I had seen on and off over the past several years. She was instrumental in helping me put my life back together after an excruciatingly painful family chasm that led to the darkest night of my soul. Concerned about my stamina, Pat urged me to cancel and reschedule. I needed to have this session. There was a lot of stuff going on in my head, and I needed to begin to sort it all out.

The thirty-minute ride was exhausting. I'm sure I must have scared the hell out of Doris when I walked into her office, even with my trusty blush and lipstick. What she saw was the true aftermath of my month-long mind-body-spirit siege. I think she might have wanted to call an ambulance. *I thought I looked pretty good…all things considered.*

We talked about my feeling that everything seemed so surreal. If what happened really happened, then I must be very powerful indeed, and that scared me. That is not how I ever saw myself, but apparently it is how others were beginning to see me. I had been in survival mode for over a month, warding off a barrage of mind-body-spirit attacks and at the same time, opening up to the miracles that saved me. Doris had steadfastly held to her belief in me and never entertained a moment of doubt that I would come through this well and whole…even better than before.

Bone-weary tired after our session, I felt more peaceful and I had a little more perspective. This was going to take some work. All in due time, I thought, but for now…rest.

Saturday, September 26, 2009

Pat took the week off to help take care of me. *What a pal!* The weekend was spent quietly. My entertainment was twice daily dressing changes and watching TV or, at least, attempting to. I would begin watching one show, fall asleep halfway through it and wake up not noticing that I was watching the latter half of a different show. Reading was not an option. I could not muster any amount of concentration. I was in a state of mental disarray or, as my mother would say, "at sixes and sevens". So I was content to catnap. I was still taking a pain pill on occasion, which I am sure significantly contributed to my semi-stuporous state.

Monday, September 28, 2009

Monday felt like a setback. I was really tired and I felt a burning sensation, like a red-hot poker, deep inside my pelvis when I stood up or walked. It felt like my bladder was on fire but not like a bladder infection. I had no fever or chills and I could pass urine without difficulty. I was to see Dr. Grace the next day. *She will fix it.*

Tuesday, September 29, 2009

Finally, I got to see Dr. Grace. She hugged me and once again expressed her joy with the outcome. I teased her about me being right and her being wrong. She agreed but then I retracted that because we were both right. She figured out what was going on and we each played our part in making it all go away.

She checked the wound and said it was healing beautifully. Of course, I told her I had an excellent home care nurse...me! Dr. Grace said the pain could be from the tissue pulling as it healed. *Fine with me.* As she was walking out the door, she stopped and cocked her head as if struck by an idea. She turned back to me and said she wanted to check something. I had learned that the head cock usually meant that I was about to dodge a bullet.

She removed the freshly-applied dressing and took a long sterile cotton swab and inserted it into my wound. She was poking around a bit and I felt a *pop.* I felt a warm, wet gush and heard her exclaim, *"Oops!"* It was a seroma. Fluid had collected and was sealed inside the wound. It felt so much better with the pressure being released. *But wait, there's more!* Dr. Grace probed deeper with the swab to discover that I had a six-inch-long "tunnel" deep underneath the surface that followed the path of the surgical incision. *Great. Now what?*

Dr. Grace announced a new game plan. She irrigated the tunnel with sterile saline and then packed it with gauze. The tunnel had to be irrigated and packed with a gauze strip twice a day to prevent further fluid buildup and to prevent infection. She wanted to order a visiting nurse to come out twice a day to do the dressing changes. I explained, having been a visiting nurse for many years, that the insurance company would not pay for that. I told her I was perfectly capable of doing it myself. She thought it would be too difficult for me given the location. Perhaps all of my nurse friends could take turns helping me. *Yeah, that's just not gonna happen.* The best way to minimize the risk of infection is to limit the number of people rendering wound care. I stubbornly and resolutely declared that I would do it myself!

The procedure was to use a syringe with a tiny flexible tube and shoot 5cc (a teaspoon) of sterile saline gently into the tunnel. After it dripped out, five feet, that's right, sixty inches of one-inch-wide packing gauze slightly dampened with saline was inserted. One end of the gauze was folded over the tip of a six-inch cotton swab and inserted up to the top of the tunnel. The remainder was inserted using the swab as a ramrod to gently insert the entire length, leaving about a one-inch tail hanging out. Over that, a saline-soaked gauze pad was placed over the entrance to the tunnel and covered with a combine. *Piece of cake.*

This would be my daily routine until the tunnel closed completely. It was imperative that the entrance to the tunnel remain open until the tunnel healed to avoid the area getting sealed off again. If that happened, it would require surgical intervention to remedy the situation.

How long was this going to take to heal? Probably several months. *We'll see about that.* For now, I will be making weekly trips to THE CANCER CENTER. When they gave me an appointment card with THE CANCER CENTER proudly displayed, I obliterated the name and wrote THE WELLNESS CENTER on it. I do not want to walk around with anything bearing the word cancer on my person or in my purse.

October 2009

I was gaining back my strength and adjusting to a new way of being. Where I was reluctant to share my story before, I couldn't stop talking about it. I would give anyone who asked how I was doing a blow-by-blow recitation of my experience. I mostly talked about how awful my whole experience was. I had been so "beaten up" by the system that I forgot to focus on my good fortune with gratitude. I had gotten away from all of the things that I had done to get to a place of healing. I had forgotten my own good advice to practice self-care. I began "tapping" again and listening to my guided imagery recordings for WellBeing. Even with that, it took some time before it felt like I got my groove back.

I was stuck in a loop of weekly visits to Dr. Grace, the hematologist, my primary care doc and the lab for blood work. I was unable to drive until the wound healed. The reason, I was told, was that if I had an accident, the steering wheel could do some major damage to my surgical area. I suggested that perhaps I could ride a motorcycle. Apparently being thrown over the handlebars could cause considerable problems as well. It was a challenge to coordinate all of the appointments and transportation. I really did not care for my dependence on others for help. I would happily drive a friend to the ends of the earth if needed and yet I felt like a burden. Still having issues with the deservedness thing. *Note to self: talk to Doris about this.*

I was able to go out socially as long as I was home by six in the evening. I was at a gathering with friends who have several dogs. I am allergic to dogs. My nose gets itchy, my eyes water and sometimes I sneeze. I hadn't considered that when I acccpted the invitation. Everything was going well. I was in a big comfy chair and I was being doted on and then it happened. Like a bolt of lightning out of the blue...I sneezed. It was one of those sneezes that originates in your toes and explodes with an atomic force. I had no time to brace myself. I saw stars. I got the whirlies. The pain ripped through me as if I had been thrown over the handlebars of a motorcycle going ninety miles an hour. Sure that my wound had expelled its entire sixty-inch streamer, I went to the bathroom to check as soon as I was able to move. Thankfully, everything was intact.

Thanks, it's been swell. Gotta go now.

CHAPTER ELEVEN

LIGHT AT THE END OF THE TUNNEL

Every week for the next thirteen weeks, I would go back to The Wellness Center to have my tunneling wound evaluated. At the fourth week, I had noticed that there were three quarter-sized hard red lumps just below my belly button. They were painful to the touch. My concern was that I had an infection in there. I returned for an emergency visit two days later. I saw the covering surgeon who cared for me in the hospital. She ordered a CT scan. I thought that was a little drastic but I guess they wanted to see definitively what was going on. The scan revealed three chambers that were inflamed at the top of the tunnel. I returned a few days later and I saw Dr. Grace, who took her trusty cotton-tipped swab and poked around a bit. This time I felt three *pops*, which released a cascade of blood-streaked purulent (pus) drainage. She prescribed two weeks of a very potent antibiotic.

I continued with my twice-daily dressing routine and the drainage quickly changed back to the usual serosanguineous drainage (clear serous fluid mixed with a little blood). Even though the infection seemed to have cleared up very nicely,

Dr. Grace ordered another week of the antibiotic. *Fine with me.*

By late November, there was still no change in the depth of the tunnel, although it had gotten somewhat narrower. Dr. Grace was beginning to think that we might need some intervention of a surgical nature. I did not warm to that idea and told her that we needed to give it a little bit more time. That evening, I was thinking about why this tunnel was not getting any smaller. As I was drifting off to sleep, it occurred to me that the tunnel could not possibly heal with the constant irritation from the packing I inserted twice daily and the slight but continuous trickle of blood caused by the blood thinners. It was also getting increasingly difficult to insert the packing because the wound opening was getting smaller and smaller. In fact, I began to use one half-inch-wide packing strips instead of the inch wide. I had also begun using the bare wooden tip of the swab because the cotton tip was too large to be inserted easily. So I decided that rather than trying to cram in several feet of the packing, I was just going to take one single eight-inch strip of the gauze and insert it, leaving only a one-inch tail sticking out so that it acted as a wick and would reduce the irritation. I only needed a small 2x2-inch gauze over the opening of the tunnel.

At my next visit, I told the nurse of my proposed plan. I did not tell her I was already doing it. She told me that it was not the protocol for tunnel wound care and I reminded her that the protocol was clearly not working. I said that I would speak with Dr. Grace about my idea. When Dr. Grace came into the examination room, after greeting me, she said a little birdie told her that I had a new plan for dealing with the tunnel. The nurse looked a little sheepish but said nothing. I told Dr. Grace that I had a talk with my body about this stubborn tunnel and she asked me what my body had to say about it. I told her what I had come up with and she thought it seemed like a reasonable idea. Then she smiled and said that there was no point in not agreeing with me because she was pretty sure I probably started to do it anyway. Indeed, I told her, I had. Lo and behold when the wound was measured after my wound care protocol, it had actually decreased by about half an inch. Dr. Grace told me to go ahead and use that plan, saying who was she to argue with my body because it hadn't failed me so far. *She really gets it now.*

The next week the tunnel had shrunk about another inch. Dr. Grace was very pleased to see the progress. After she left, Baby Doc stopped in to say hello. I had not seen her since before surgery, although she was in the OR, but I was asleep. She wanted to tell me how happy she was at the good outcome of the pathology. I told her that my thoughts changed my DNA and that the cancer just left my body and that I worked very hard to make it all go away. I did, of course, give mega props to the docs, and I meant that sincerely. She then pondered aloud that although it was highly unlikely, that despite all of the pre-op findings, it could still be in the realm of possibility that there was no cancer to begin with. *She just wasn't gonna let this one go.* So I cupped my ear with my hand and said, "Shh. What's that I hear?" She looked at me quizzically and said she didn't hear anything. I jokingly said, "Oh that's the sound of your mind slamming shut." She took my humor (sarcasm) in good stride and I told her that I did appreciate her good wishes. I had been through so much and I was really amping up my authenticity about who I had become. *I could no longer just nod my head and pretend none of this happened the way it did. Nope, not anymore.*

So here we were at week thirteen of the tunnel saga. It was December 23rd. I really wanted to get sprung from the weekly visits for the Christmas holidays. Dr. Grace had told me that if the tunnel was closed adequately, she would spring me for two weeks. By now I was able to insert only about an inch to an inch and a half of the packing plus the little tail hanging out. The bleeding and drainage was virtually nil. Happily, Dr. Grace agreed that it was just about closed and she would be comfortable not seeing me for two weeks. Yippee! I joked that I would have nothing to look forward to after the New Year. She said we were going to start the New Year off by repeating that CA125 and she would be doing my first post-op pelvic exam. *Great. Can't wait.*

She had been putting off repeating the CA125, the marker for ovarian cancer, because things like the trauma of surgery or an infection could yield a false high reading. So we had to wait until I was fully recovered from surgery, the wound was completely healed, and of course the infection was no longer an issue. I actually looked forward to having the CA125 repeated. After all, everything was gone, so why wouldn't it be back to normal? The internal exam, not so much.

During this time I would be asked the same list of questions at each visit. The answers, I am sure, were to glean a snapshot of my progress. However, there was no additional probing regardless of my responses. There seemed to be no other purpose other than filling out the forms. These questions were clearly geared toward someone who was in active treatment for cancer, which I was not. So much of it was irrelevant in my case. Other than that cursed tunnel, the rest of me was doing well.

I took umbrage with some of the information gathering. Every visit, the tech asked me to get on the scale. Not being high on my list of favorite things to do and not seeing the significance of providing this information in my case, I began to refuse. I was told by the tech that I "had to" get on the scale. I replied that it was privileged information. She said that she would get into trouble if she didn't fill in all the blanks. I told her to just write down "fat". She said she couldn't write that down. So just write down, "kinda fat" or "pleasingly plump". That did not go over well. Then just write down "patient refused". That seemed to assuage her somewhat.

Then they wanted to take my blood pressure. My blood pressure was always within normal limits at home, however, with my documented White Coat Syndrome, my readings were always elevated in a doctor's office. I saw my primary care doctor regularly to have the blood thinners monitored and he monitored my blood pressure as well. The nurse intervened to say that it was a necessary part of my care. I asked what they would do about it if I had high blood pressure and she said that I should see my primary care doctor. So I told her what I told the tech, write down "patient refused".

I was asked about my level of energy and I responded that it was pretty low. I asked what they could do about it and I was told to get plenty of rest. *Gee, now why didn't I think of that?*

The nurse asked if I was sexually active. Nope. *Seriously? Nothing says sexy like a gaping hole between your belly button and your hoo-hah with a little white tail hanging out of it.* I did have a little fun with them as they continued to ask about the status of my sexual (or lack thereof) activity each week. *No, I just lay there. Do you have anyone in mind? Does it count if I'm by myself? Not according to Bill Clinton.*

I bring this up because it is an important issue for all women who have undergone GYN surgery with or without cancer. *Is it safe to have sex? Will it hurt? Will everything work like it did before? Will it be mutually satisfying? Will the drive ever come back? Do I want it to come back?* Many women may have had no sex drive for a period of time leading up to the diagnosis and treatment. *Am I still desirable? Have I lost my femininity?* Women may grieve the loss of their ability to bear children.

I certainly could have asked any question about any issues I felt were pressing, but I just wanted to get back to my life. I would encourage any woman and her spouse or partner to ask any questions that are of concern and to speak with a mental health professional to help sort out the myriad of issues that will inevitably come up.

The one question I did ask was what happened to the space where everything was removed? I guess I should have known the answer, but I wanted to be sure that nothing could get lost in the abyss. The remaining tissue, muscle, ligaments and fat fill in the void and the vagina is closed off like a blind pouch. I was assured that it was quite commodious. *Good to know should anyone ask.*

Being my last visit before the Christmas holidays, I brought in a couple of trays of bagels with assorted cream cheeses. Big hit. Nurses love to be fed. They were grateful that it wasn't another tray of cookies and candies. As I was leaving, one of the nurses commented that I must be happy to put this year behind me. I told her that despite the challenges, it ended up to be a very good year. I didn't have cancer anymore, my wound was closed, my WellBeing was restored and my mother was finally at peace.

Life is good.

CHAPTER TWELVE

HOME STRETCH

I was delighted to have only one visit to my primary care doctor to have my Coumadin level checked and one trip to the hospital over the holidays to have some blood work done. Funny how only two health care visits seemed like a vacation.

Christmas was spent quietly with friends. I was amazed that I was able to do all of my Christmas shopping online and even found a few bargains in the process. Mall shopping has never been a favorite activity for me.

Still recouping my strength and having a lot of time on my hands, I was totally *bored out of my gourd*. I had never been one for crafts, however, I found myself drawn to one particular crafty activity which I learned about two summers ago while attending The Humor Project conference at Lake George in New York State. It is such a positive, openhearted and uproariously fun three days. Another attendee had given me this very simple and useful bookmark crafted from a piece of string with colorful beads on each end. She called it a book thong, as it was placed in the crack of your book to hold your place. I loaded up on supplies from a local craft store and made everyone I knew – friends, the mailman, the

UPS guy and neighbors – a personalized book thong using alphabet beads to spell out their name. The boredom problem was solved. *Ah, but I digress.* They were, by the way, a big hit.

Never being one to ring in the New Year with any fanfare, I had dinner with friends and then home in bed by nine o'clock. My personal year in review was quite the roller coaster ride. My New Year's resolution was to find a way to share my experience with others and to empower them to embrace their own abilities for self-healing. Now I just had to figure out exactly what I did and how I did it and I'd be on my way. Turned out not to be such an easy task.

As much physical healing that had taken place, the emotional and spiritual parts of my journey were far from over. I continued to see Doris regularly and to have Reiki sessions with Roxie. I also treated myself to relaxing yet gentle massages every week. I recognized that I needed to practice self-care to maintain a continued sense of Wellbeing.

Having received a generous inheritance after my mother's passing, I was able to take the next year off to regroup and still have a financial cushion. *Who knew my father had been such a whiz kid in the stock market?*

This made it possible for me not to have to return to my soul-sucking job. I believe with all my heart and soul that if I had to go back to a job that was not in alignment with who I had become and did not move me in the direction of my ever-emerging life purpose, it would have been more devastating to my health and WellBeing than any disease known to man. I was feeling truly blessed on so many levels.

January 6, 2010

I had a nine o'clock appointment with the Dr. Cleary, the hematologist. I don't know why they schedule an appointment that early when the doctor doesn't even get there until ten-thirty or eleven and nothing can be done beyond vital signs, which I refused anyway. Around ten o'clock, the hematology Fellow of the month came in, which is usual.

This one looked through my chart and seemed more interested in the cancer part than the blood clot part. After reviewing my blood work and history, he asked me if I was finished with my chemo. I told him that I did not have chemo. He said, "Are you sure you didn't have chemo?" *Hmmm. Let me think about this. Yep, I'm sure.* He was incredulous that with a CA125 of 17,000 that I didn't need chemo. *Even though I have referenced this number earlier, this was the first time I became aware of that actual number. I am glad that I had steadfastly refused to know the numbers before. That would have gotten into my nurse brain and scared the hell out of me.* He kept expressing his incredulity about me not having chemo and I told him that I didn't need it because after surgery, there was nothing to treat. I told him that I was cancer free, which is a term I never use. I just don't feel the need to define myself by a disease I no longer have.

He looked me squarely in the eye and said, "Yes, you are cancer free...for now." This guy was hell-bent on messing with my head, so I looked him squarely in the eye and said, "Yes and you are cancer free too...for now." I could tell he did not like having *his* head messed with. *How do you like me now?* He then told me (*not asked*) to hop (*yeah right!*) up on the table so he could examine me. He gave me the creeps. I felt like a lab rat. *No. You may not examine me. Why? I don't like you, now please go away.*

Dr. Cleary came in without the Fellow and made no mention of him. She, too, struggled with my outcome because the numbers, my medical history and the pathology just didn't line up with what one would expect. I had told her from day one, as I did anyone with whom I spoke, that I was going to make this all go away. That just did not compute with her academic bent, however, she never challenged me, for which I am grateful. She was anxious to know the CA125 results, which had been greatly delayed because of the wound infection. I asked about getting the filters out since I was not having chemo and the cancer was gone. After we see the CA125, which would be drawn the following week. *Fine!*

Late January, 2010

The big day had arrived, or so it was for Dr. Grace. Although I did not have to go through any more wound and dressing rigmarole, I would have my first post-op internal exam and Pap smear. I would also get the results of the CA125 that was drawn prior to the visit. I was happy about the wound being a thing of the past despite the fact that the resulting scar was a bit horrifying to behold. I had no sense of anticipation for the test results except where Dr. Cleary and getting the filters out were concerned. The internal exam was another story. I asked Dr. Grace if we could just go out to lunch. She chuckled and said that doing a pelvic exam might be a little awkward in a crowded restaurant. It's good to have a doctor with a sense of humor.

All was well as expected as far as I was concerned. She was jubilant when she announced that the CA 125 was...wait for it...11, perfectly within normal range. Pretty impressive now that I knew what the original number was, the number that the medical student was about to reveal to me right before his banishment. *Little pissant!*

Dr. Grace and I had this running joke that with each milestone, I would ask, "Did you expect anything less from me?" She would always say, "From you? No." She told me, however, that she had hoped for a slow and gradual decrease of the CA125 and revealed that she had rarely seen such a high number. She was not expecting it to come down so low and so quickly. I reminded her that this might be true for mere mortals. I asked Dr. Grace if she would speak with Dr. Cleary since she was dragging her feet about letting me have the filters taken out. She said that she may be less concerned now that the CA125 is normal.

It was time to discuss the follow-up plan. Her plan was for check-ups every three months for the first two years and then every six months for the next three years with a Pap smear and a CA125 with each visit. Additionally, I was to have a CT scan in three months and then every six months to a year. I asked why so many visits, so often and why the CT scans? It was the standard protocol. She admitted that was the protocol for someone undergoing cancer treatment. *But what do you do for a patient like me?* Apparently, she had never had a patient quite like me.

It was clear that I was not a standard kind of gal, so we needed to negotiate a nonstandard plan. I agreed to visits every three months for year one, every six months for year two and once a year thereafter and no CT scans. I was not going to agree to be exposed to radiation for a cancer hunt. While Dr. Grace was supportive and open to my unique situation, she was still a scientist. I respected her perspective as she respected mine. I told her how much I appreciated her support and compassion as well her skills as a surgeon. Strange as it seems, I knew I would miss our weekly visits.

Some months later, it occurred to me that the wound would not heal because it was my only way of staying connected with Dr. Grace, with whom I shared what I felt was a strong spiritual bond. When I was at a point where I could integrate and align my mind, body and spirit in harmony, I could let go. When I finally let go, the wound healed quickly. I was given a three-month pass.

Time to cut the cord.

CHAPTER THIRTEEN

PUMPING IRON

Early February, 2010

Settling into a routine continued to be an issue. Unless your idea of a routine is a doctor visit once or twice a week. Ever since surgery, my Coumadin levels had been difficult to stabilize even though I was meticulous to avoid foods that could increase or decrease my clotting times. Certain foods can cause your blood to become "thin" or clot too slowly, increasing the risk of bleeding heavily from a cut or injury. Other foods can cause your blood to clot too fast, and I've already been down that road. These foods are of no concern to someone who does not have a clotting disorder.

Although standard blood tests revealed only slight anemia, I continued to complain of severe fatigue. Despite taking massive amounts of iron supplements, more in-depth blood tests showed that I had very low (almost nonexistent) Ferritin (iron store) levels. Dr. Cleary, who resumed charge of my care after getting out of the hospital, expressed concern that there may be some hidden bleeding in my GI tract or elsewhere. The unspoken concern was that there might be a new blood-sucking tumor lurking somewhere in my body. I had already been scoped, scanned, poked, prodded, pricked and sliced and diced, and I was clean. *Nope, not goin' down that road again!*

The concern was reasonable from the doctor's point of view, however, I had no such concerns as I had spent all of my teen and adult years dealing with anemia due to a myriad of GYN issues, and I believed that it was going to take some time to regain my hemodynamic equilibrium, that is, to give my body time to adjust to all of the changes.

Dr. Cleary suggested that I have another colonoscopy and endoscopy done to rule out any hidden bleeding. I declined. She then suggested that I have intravenous iron infusions since the massive amounts of iron supplements proved to be inadequate. This requires five infusions of iron over a period of ten days to two weeks. It had to be done at the hospital and I wanted to get them five days in a row to get it over with as quickly as possible. She agreed.

I was scheduled for the infusions for the next week. I was surprised and more than a little rattled when I entered the infusion unit. The sign on the door read, "Same Day Chemo Unit". I had no issue being in a room with patients receiving chemo. It's just that I was still adjusting on some level to not having cancer. While the non-cancer patients were few and far between, I just didn't see the need for the ubiquitous cancer signage being shoved down my throat.

In preparation for the iron infusion, I was pre-medicated with 50 mg of Benadryl (in case of an allergic reaction). Twenty-five mg of Benadryl can put me into a semi-coma, so 50 mg put me into major La-La Land. The infusion ran over a couple of hours and then I was hydrated with more IV fluids afterwards. Having had all of my veins used up during my surgical days, starting an IV proved to be difficult for these nurses, who are the best of the best IV starters.

My plan to have five infusions in a row was aborted after the first infusion. After returning home in midafternoon, I napped. When I awakened, I felt as if I had been run over by an eighteen wheeler. A little change in plans was in order. I opted for the two week plan.

One more hurdle.

CHAPTER FOURTEEN

UNFILTERED

Late February, 2010

---

had my follow up visit with Dr. Cleary after the iron infusions. My blood work was good and I was cut loose for six weeks. Any questions? *About those filters?* Still hedging around, Dr. Cleary cautioned that the filters may not be able to be removed since they had been in for so long. I knew we were down to the wire time-wise. They had been in for five months and the magic number was six months. Complicating things was that there were two filters in place. One that went in through the groin and had to be removed via the neck and the other inserted through the neck and needed to come out through the groin. They could already be stuck if the lining of the vessel grew around them. *Tricky but not impossible. Besides, who do you think you're dealing with here? I'm Nurse Crilly, self-healing machine. 'Nuf said!*

I suggested that if the interventional radiologist (IR) put his foot in my groin and gave a good yank, it would probably come right out. *Just kidding...maybe.* Finally she agreed to speak with the IR about it.

I received a call from Dr. Cleary's office that I was scheduled for an ultrasound to check the location of the filters (they can travel) and the status of the offending blood clot which can also travel. The clot needed to be "organized"; that is, it must be sealed over and adhered to the side of the vessel wall without danger of breaking loose.

I would need to call upon my healing mojo once again. I focused on there being no clot at all. I focused on a clean, smooth vessel wall. I continued to focus on my WellBeing.

Ultrasound Day
March 1, 2010

I reported to the outpatient ultrasound department and was led to a little dark room and instructed to lay on the stretcher. A very sweet and very young ultrasound tech explained the procedure and she began to move the rather chilly ultrasound wand up and down the center of my abdomen. I could see the screen but it looked like static to me. After about ten minutes, she excused herself and returned with a slightly older and presumably more seasoned tech. The new tech repeated the process and I could see that there was an issue. Finally, one said that she identified the filter. I mentioned that there were two. Nope, we just see one. Are you sure you have two filters? *As sure I as I am that I didn't have chemo. Yes, I'm sure.*

I asked if they identified the clot. Not yet. The clot had been sandwiched in between the two filters. Both techs left and moments later returned with another machine. Cold wand to the tummy again. *Anything?* They found the two filters where they should have been but still no sign of the clot. *Maybe it's gone?* No, that just doesn't happen. I told them that I made it go away just like I made the cancer go away. They laughed uncomfortably and left the room again. I got off the table to spy on them. They were on the phone with Dr. Rand, the interventional radiologist who put in the second filter.

They returned shortly for a fourth pass. This time they were moving the wand right and left over my abdomen. This seemed odd to me, as they were nowhere near where the clot was located, but since they could not find it, Dr. Rand said to check the renal (kidney) and hepatic (liver) veins to see if it had migrated. Nope, not there either. At a loss, they said that they must speak to the doctor again but not to worry. *Who's worried?*

Again I eavesdropped on the conversation. The senior tech was getting an earful from the doctor. She laughed nervously as she told the doctor that I said that I made the clot disappear. They never did find the clot and I was free to leave. Whatever the doc saw or didn't see on the ultrasound, it was good enough for him to schedule removal of the filters. *Finally!*

March 3, 2010

I was admitted to the same day surgery area at seven a.m. I was excited and curious as to how this could be accomplished because of the crisscross situation with the filters. I was brought down to the IR unit where my stretcher was parked in the narrow hallway. Dr. Rand, with his impish grin and disarming manner, came to talk to me. He explained that the filters had been in for a long time and...blah, blah, blah. He said he would try his best to get them out. I told him that *try* implies the possibility of failure and that he must believe that he would be successful. I said that they would slip out like *buttah*. I told him no drama like last time. Just knock me out and yank out those filters!

After two hours, I awakened to have Dr. Rand tell me, excitedly, that both filters did indeed slip out like *buttah* and that he found no evidence of the clot. It was as if it had never been there. If he had not seen it himself in the first place, he would not have believed it. He shook his head and marveled at my "positive attitude".

And the miracles just keep on comin'.

PART TWO

CHAPTER FIFTEEN

WHY DID I GET CANCER?

I get asked that question a lot. I am also frequently asked the unanswerable "why me" question. It seems as if they want to know what I did or didn't do to get cancer. This stems from the fear on the part of the questioner and they want to ascertain, and not in a pejorative way, where my failure came from. Was it a religious shortcoming? Something I ate or drank too much or too little of? A cancer diagnosis brings out strong feelings of blame, shame and guilt. Some of it, I confess, was self-inflicted. I felt like my body had betrayed me and that made me very angry. To add insult to injury, it was the core of my womanhood that turned against me. I began to think of my reproductive organs as a separate entity. They became my enemy even though I never abused them. Hell, not having had children, I never even used them! This betrayal began long ago. I had a history of gynecological issues since my late teens marked by many months of amenorrhea (no period) followed by longer stretches of menorrhagia (prolonged periods of extreme heavy bleeding) that could only be controlled by mega doses of birth control pills. There were also the not infrequent hemorrhages that required a D&C. I had nine of them plus five uterine biopsies, many without anesthesia due to the emergent nature of the blood loss. *Ouch!*

The pathology was always benign but with each negative result came the same warning. "If this bleeding continues, you will need a hysterectomy." By the time I was in my early forties, I didn't give a rat's ass. *Take it out. Take it all out!* Then the warnings became, "If you keep taking these hormone pills...**YOU ARE GOING TO GET CANCER!**" *Then stop prescribing the pills and take out my uterus. Rip it out. I don't need it!* The response was always the same. I had a healthy uterus and they didn't want to take out a healthy organ. *Great! So let's just wait until I get cancer or bleed to death.* This was the message I received over and over for nearly forty years from at least a dozen gynecologists. They scolded me as if I was doing something wrong or not doing something right to cause this. I felt tremendous shame as if I was less than what a women should be. It struck at the very heart of my femininity. I felt guilty that I couldn't do more or be more. If I knew then what I know now, I could have and would have done something to heal my body and my spirit. *I also would have told those doctors to kiss my ass!*

In 1998, I had what was then a brand new procedure called an endometrial ablation (I called it the Boil 'N Bag procedure). A balloon was inserted into my uterus and filled with water that was then heated to nearly the boiling point and the inside of the uterine walls (the endometrium) were, essentially, scalded. The outcome was that the resulting scar tissue made it (luckily, in my case) nearly impossible to produce a menstrual flow. That ended the bleeding and the need for the hormone pills. I was finally free except for occasional spotting until I reached a natural menopause two years later. I was happy to finally be feeling well and yet at the same time I grieved the loss of my ability to bear a child.

At the age of forty-six there was no hope or desire to become pregnant but having the choice taken away from me and the finality of it was painful nonetheless. I was no longer plagued by the severe fatigue-inducing anemia and my subsequent Pap smears were normal. I assumed I was out of the woods. *Guess again.*

I received persistent messages of an impending and inevitable diagnosis of GYN cancer over that forty-year period. That does not really answer the question as to why I got cancer, however, the groundwork for the possibility was laid. It was a message that was played over and over again externally by the doctors and internally by the little voice in my head. On some level, I believed cancer was inevitable. Remember, beliefs are thoughts we keep thinking. They got in my head. If only I had known the influence and power of these messages, I am sure things would have turned out differently. I am not suggesting that I gave myself cancer. The implication, however, was clear that I did little to prevent it.

The Blame Game

I was not living a healthy lifestyle by any stretch of the imagination. I gave no heed to the stresses of my career path as a nurse. I was a bit of an adrenalin junkie back in the day, preferring the fast-paced life and death drama of the neonatal intensive care unit caring for very sick and extremely premature infants. It was rewarding but it took its toll physically and emotionally. Among my other jobs was as executive director of a start-up children's hospice. This was rewarding work as well but emotionally draining, even devastating at times. I was also a pediatric visiting nurse in a crime-ridden and poverty-stricken urban area where shoot-outs, drug deals and car hijackings were the order of the day. I was a two pack a day smoker and a home cooked meal consisted of heating up fast food in the microwave. This lack of self-care was a contributing factor to cracking open the window of opportunity for disease to creep in by lowering my overall emotional and physical health, especially my immune system. I blamed myself and I felt tremendous shame. Many healthcare practitioners laid blame as well while piling on a heaping dose of shame because as a nurse, I should have taken better care of myself. The shame and blame from myself and others brought out the Catholic guilts with a vengeance. All of those "if onlys" and all of the "coulda, shoulda, wouldas" I berated myself with were a complete waste of valuable time and energy.

I guess you could say that I allowed myself, unwittingly, to become a *hospitable host*. I repeat, this does not in any way, shape or form suggest that I gave myself cancer. I did not allow it in. I did not invite it in. I sure as hell did not welcome it in. I was just ripe for the pickin's.

As much as I embrace a philosophy and a belief system that supports self-healing and as much as I cherish the relationships that have developed among my like-thinking friends and colleagues, I have received unwanted messages from this group as well. Certainly not the vast majority. These folks are really kind hearted and well meaning. There are some, however, whose blame and shame philosophy were equally as harmful as the traditionalists. In sharing what I thought was a beautiful story of healing and self-discovery, I would inevitably be confronted by some who would ask me why I allowed the cancer in. What lesson did I need to learn? What message was I ignoring that I needed cancer in order to get my attention? There were certainly many takeaways and enlightenment from my experience, however, I don't think I was being punished with cancer for not learning my lessons sooner or for not paying attention to the messages. From the rest of the "woo-woo" crowd, I received many kudos and well wishes.

Illness as a Metaphor

Putting the shame, blame and guilt aside, I believ illness and disease mirror what is going on in our lives. As said before, disease is opportunistic. It will seek out the weak spot in our armor. We are inextricably intertwined emotionally, physically and spiritually. A chink in our emotional armor can manifest itself physically. For example, one might develop chronic stomach pain or migraines after a traumatic event or experiencing a persistently high level of stress. A physical chink can create an emotional disruption, such as, an injury that is temporarily or permanently disabling releasing a cascade of negative emotions. These are generalities, of course.

In a metaphorical sense, consider the person with chronic neck pain. I bet you would hear him refer to people on a regular basis as being a "pain in the neck". Here is a true story and a cautionary tale about negative self-talk. Back in 1999 when I was just beginning to go public with my holistic wellness leanings, I worked with a nurse, Carla, who had the most negative attitude I have ever encountered. If you looked up "negative attitude" in the dictionary, you would see her picture there. I will admit that her personal life was filled with stress, as she bore the huge responsibility of being a single mom taking care of a severely handicapped adult child.

Every day, when she came into the office where I worked as a nursing supervisor, you could feel the energy get sucked right out of the room. Even before she hung up her coat, she was off and running about her difficult commute, all the work she had to do that day and all the stupid people she would have to deal with. Her job was no picnic but she NEVER...EVER let up! I noticed that for the previous week or so, she had been complaining that her stomach was "tied up in knots". We've all had that feeling at one time or another, however, this was constant. I told her that she

etting a handle on her stress and that I
help her with some stress management
:ked together for about half an hour at
.tted that her stomach felt better and her
ιe from a ten plus to about a five. I asked
o lower it further. Her answer surprised
me anu, զ--   kly, shocked me when she said no. When I
inquired as to why she wanted to hold on to that much stress
after seeing how quickly and easily she let it go, she replied,
"If I let all of my stress go, I won't know who I am anymore".
Phew! That was a new one on me but something I have seen
many times since. When you invite people to step out of
their belief comfort zone even when it is in their highest
good, it can create tremendous anxiety.

That very evening, Carla was rushed to the hospital with
severe abdominal pain that required emergency surgery. The
diagnosis was a volvulus, which happens when the large
intestines get twisted up and compress the blood supply,
causing horrific pain and damage to the bowel. Her guts
were, quite literally, "tied up in knots". She rather accurately
pinpointed the source of the physical manifestation of her
emotional stress. *Coincidence? I don't think so.*

I don't know which comes first, the metaphor or the
belief. Is the metaphor the precursor to an illness or is it the
persistent thought that creates the illness? It may be both.
Either way, it all contributes to the cascading effects of our
thoughts on our health.

CHAPTER SIXTEEN

WHAT'S YOUR SIGN?

Cancer is one of the most powerful and fear-provoking words in the English language – or any language for that matter. Just the mere mention of the word cancer causes a visceral response. It hits you right in the gut. When I told my mother that my youngest sister, Jean, had been diagnosed with uterine cancer at the age of thirty-eight, she clutched her abdomen and took several steps back. Always tightly in control in the face of a crisis, her immediate response was unsettling for me to witness. After reassuring her, as best I could, that Jean would be in good hands with an excellent Gynecologist/Oncologist, she relaxed a bit. She said it felt as if she had been punched in the stomach by a heavyweight boxer. Fortunately, the cancer was Stage I and Jean required no further treatment after surgery. There were some people, upon hearing her prognosis, who said she was lucky because she had the "good" kind of cancer. *Didn't know there was such a thing.* That was nearly twenty years ago and Jean has long since been given a clean bill of health. It was because of the frightened reaction of friends and family members to Jean's news that I decided not to share more information about my situation than was necessary.

When I was going through the whole cancer process, there was no escaping that word, certainly not at THE CANCER CENTER or THE CANCER HOSPITAL. That word was everywhere: on all of the literature, appointment cards, lab coat breast pockets, the posters and pamphlets and yes, let us not forget that rainbow assortment of ribbons.

Cancer doesn't even have a decent nickname or code word. In medicine we call it "CA". In layman's language it is referred to as the big "C". I refuse to give it such elevated status. I prefer little "c". If I never had to use that word again, I wouldn't. When speaking to groups, I begin my story with, "In 2009, I was diagnosed with invasive ovarian cancer..." I can see in the faces of the audience a mix of sadness, deep empathy and fear. Their body language conveys the same message. Often, I hear a collective drawn out "oh" with the inflection going way down at the end. This is a heck of a way to start a humorous and uplifting presentation, but I like to get it out of the way right up front.

When it comes up in conversation, the overwhelmingly most popular response is "I'm so sorry". I tell them not to be sorry because I'm fine. Many times, though we met as strangers, upon hearing my story, they will spontaneously give me a hug. A good hug. A great big happy hug, not a sad or scared hug.

That "cancer" word is so powerful, it seems like it is a living breathing entity from the dark side. How did it get to be so powerful? We did it. Perhaps because way back when, there was little that could be offered in traditional medicine to treat it and it was more often than not a death sentence. Let's be honest here. Emphysema, diabetes and heart disease are no picnic either. I imagine that given a choice of cancer or the aforementioned diseases, nobody would pick cancer.

Here's my point. It is the fear of the word cancer almost as much as the disease itself that makes it so powerful. It is the fear that causes the cascade of immune-suppressing stress responses when faced with cancer or even the possibility of it. It is the fear mongering of the media that fuels the fire. Just simply speaking the word cancer, hearing it or reading it elicits the fight, flight or freeze response. I am not lying when I say that the word has always scared the bejesus out of me and still does, just not quite as much anymore. It mostly annoys the shit out of me now. I'd like to tell you that cancer is just a word like any other word, but I would be lying. I had to do some major soul searching and work on healing my energy around the word to be okay with the subtitle of this book.

So frightful did I find the word cancer that I counted myself as quite lucky not to have been born prematurely of my mid-August expected date of arrival, which would have made my birth under the sign of Cancer. Please take no offense you warm-hearted, gentle souls born under this sign, for none was intended. I guess I was destined to be born under the sign of the Lion and not the Crab because I truly am such a Leo at heart.

I believe I may have come up with a solution for that "c" word. I have given this great thought. I was pondering one day during my convalescence that there must be a better word that does not release the Kraken of Fear. And then it hit me. How much less frightening would it be if instead of hearing, "We have completed all the tests and I am sorry to say that you have cancer", the doctor would say, "We have completed all the tests and you have crabs!" *Kind of takes the wind out of the sails a bit, don't you think?*

I have since stopped using the "c" word after the initial sharing of my story and have replaced it with "crabs". It has led to some very interesting situations over the years. I was with a few colleagues and casually referred back to when I had crabs and everyone took it with aplomb except for a newbie to the group, who audibly gasped as she leaned way back in her seat, getting as far away from me as possible. Another time, a woman sitting near my table in a crowded café apparently overheard part of my explanation to my friend about having had ovarian crabs. After a few minutes, she tapped me on the shoulder and asked where I got Bavarian crabs, to which I replied, "From a Bavarian, of course."

CHAPTER SEVENTEEN

WHAT'S GOD GOT TO DO WITH IT?

Having read Part One and assuming that you didn't skip ahead, I am sure the questions that came to mind were "What did you do to heal yourself?" Or "How did you do it?" The answer is both simple and at the same time quite complex. I will answer those questions and many more that have been asked of me as I shared my story with groups and individuals. The reason I waited four years to get started on this book was because it took me that long to figure some things out.

Let me be clear about one thing from the get go. When I speak of healing myself or use the term self-healing in general, I have often been criticized for leaving God out of the equation. Although I was raised Catholic, I do not embrace any particular religion. I do, however, take from many faiths those ideas and ideals that resonate with me. I am a deeply spiritual person with a belief that at the core of all things is a Higher Power, Source Energy, All-That-Is or whatever politically correct term one cares to attach to the concept of God.

The God of the Catholic teachings in the '50s and '60s never sat well with me, and I often questioned the paradox that an omnipotent and all-loving God could banish to Limbo an infant who died before being baptized. Limbo didn't sound like it would be much fun for anyone, much less a baby. My ten-year-old self questioned the good Sister Theresa (her name was changed to spare me from eternal damnation) about this whole Limbo thing. I suggested that God would just pop the baby's barely used soul into another new baby as it made its way into the world. Well, apparently the notion of recycled souls or reincarnation, if you prefer, was a no-no and earned me the rank of heretic and blasphemer, for which I was appropriately humiliated and chastised. It left me confused and angry and although I continued my Catholic education through high school and attended a Catholic nursing school, my faith was an empty shell. There was one small nugget of belief that I secretly held on to for all these years. My favorite teacher, Mr. Frank Schoenig, who taught seventh and eighth grade science, offered proof as to the existence of God. He said that looking back to the origin of time and space there was a Prime Mover. I am paraphrasing (hey, it's been fifty years) by saying that there was an energetic force that had to get the ball rolling in the first place and that would be God. I later learned that idea was from the teachings of Aristotle and later, St. Thomas Aquinas. I was able to live with that and it had always held me in great stead.

I believe in the power of prayer or as some call it, the Law of Attraction. I believe in Angels as messengers from the Universe. I don't believe that there is a hell nor do I believe in a vengeful God who, indiscriminately, metes out punishment to us souls who are having a human experience. I do believe, however, that there is a heaven, each of us creating our own version of it.

Religion tends to personify God and Angels by attributing human emotions, logic and judgment. I think this diminishes our capacity to draw from the tremendous and powerful resources available to us from the Universe and it puts limitations on our potential as human beings. My vision of God is as an energetic presence that is pure love. Relating to God and Angels with human characteristics make it easier for us to wrap our heads around the enormity and profundity of what we are capable of understanding in the dimension or realm in which we now exist. *Wow, deep, huh?*

I have become comfortable again using the "G" word or other synonyms of Divine reference without fear of sounding like a religious zealot to agnostics, atheists or nihilists. The most important thing that I learned in defining my relationship with God was that we are not separate entities. We truly are all One. I believe God is seamlessly interwoven into the matrix of all things. And here is the kicker. So are we all. When I say that I healed myself, it is implicit that I did not do this alone. I had help from Source and the Universal connectedness we all share.

I have heard so often over the years, patients and their families saying in despair, "It's in God's hands now." That is true, however, God's hands are your hands. I always felt that these words were said by those who gave up or felt powerless. You do not need to give up or give over control, responsibility or hope in order to receive Divine intervention. Praying for a miracle is a good thing, however, I believe that we must be active participants through our thoughts, beliefs and actions. When I embraced the belief that God is an internal source and not an external source, I felt the true power of my "self". Some may ask what difference this makes. The difference is that I see myself as the captain of my own ship (free will) and God is my navigator (Divine Guidance).

This experience forced me to take a good hard look at my beliefs. Not just religion or faith, but my beliefs around health, healing, happiness, deservedness, worthiness, love, prosperity and abundance. My whole world was turned upside down and I had to struggle to figure out which way was up.

I do not claim to have all the answers or even most of them when it comes to matters of God, life or the Universe at large. You don't have to sign on to my beliefs to be healed or to be healthy. I offer my philosophy as something to ponder or as something you may wish to consider in its entirety or piecemeal. Or put together what feels right for you. The important thing is that whatever beliefs you cling to, make sure that they are serving your highest good.

CHAPTER EIGHTEEN

DECONSTRUCTION ZONE

Many have asked for my healing recipe. I was still nursing my post-op incision and people were already encouraging me to write a book about my healing – a "how to" book. This is not that book. At least that was not my intention. I thought it was important to share the chronology of my journey and to bear witness to the miracles that punctuated every step of the way.

I made no bones about the nontraditional way in which I sought healing. I am acutely aware that the path I chose to walk might have been considered "out there" and a little too woo-woo for many, especially those in the medical community, and I'm okay with that. There was still enough of the traditionalist in me as a nurse not to turn my back on conventional medicine. This was due, in part, to the fact that I had no fully executable Plan A of my own. However, I never let the strictly allopathic Plan A interfere with my grand scheme of ultimate WellBeing nor did I find it necessary to interfere with theirs. *Okay, well maybe a little.*

I must emphatically state that I would never encourage anyone to dismiss out of hand any treatment options, whether they come from traditional medicine or the alternative healing arts. There were those who strongly chastised me for "selling out" by having surgery. I would have happily skipped that part of the program, however, my body was severely compromised by the presence of the huge tumor that was compressing the veins in my legs which caused the blood clots. I did not feel that I had the luxury of time to wait any longer, and at the same time I acknowledged that this was a pre-programmed self-limiting belief. Following their argument, I also should have done more in terms of self-care to help prevent the whole thing in the first place. That may be true, however, I was dealing in the present, and after taking everything into account, I did what I was guided to do, what my gut told me to do. In retrospect, I think that I may have been a little more proactive and waited a couple of weeks before surgery because the signs of healing were coming fast and furious and I now believe that I would have been completely healed of all evidence that cancer was there. I was afraid at the time to even broach this subject with anyone. My advice would be that unless you are in a life-threatening situation, take a little time, perhaps a couple of days or a week to consider your options and get all of your allopathic and holistic healing ducks in a row.

The truth is that I initially thought that I would have, with great reluctance, gone the whole chemo/radiation route, if necessary. After the *knowing,* I could comfortably keep that as a back burner option, secure in believing that my complete wellness would still be the ultimate outcome. Each of us is on our own unique path and how we traverse the terrain is always our choice. I chose to take as much control over my WellBeing and to remain as true to my authentic self as possible while maintaining some sense of balance with my allopathic leanings as a nurse. *It wasn't easy.*

Many applauded my bravery while claiming their own lack of courage should they ever be faced with a devastating diagnosis such as mine. I was placed on a pedestal and, uncomfortably, held in great esteem for this, and I always found it perplexing. I can only say that I did not think that there was anything brave or courageous about choosing to live and be well. While I eschewed the idea of being courageous, I am willing to cop to dogged (read stubborn) determination and a goodly dose of fortitude.

I cannot give you a blueprint for healing, however, each chapter in Part II of this book was written to deconstruct the process that made my healing possible. Admittedly, I used the "kitchen sink" approach, throwing in every aspect of healing the mind, body and spirit that I could come up with. This plan was scattershot, disorganized, untested and unproven. And yet...it worked. To be clear, it was not the techniques by themselves that healed me. It was not the practitioners who healed me (none of them ever claimed that they did). My body healed itself. With the help of friends and colleagues, Angels, the God within me and yes, the doctors and nurses too, my body was able to heal itself. By redirecting energy via my thoughts, my emotions and my beliefs, my body received the proper information it needed to self-repair. No magic, just science, pure and simple. How I got here is where the magic came in. The point where science meets spirit.

CHAPTER NINETEEN

BELIEVE IT OR NOT!

In Chapter One, I mentioned that in order to release the fear, I needed to change my belief about cancer being a death sentence. Thankfully, I was able to do that rather quickly, although I did run into one wall after another of negative self-limiting beliefs that were standing in the way of my being well and whole.

Let's delve a little deeper into this whole belief thing. Your core beliefs make you "who you are", or so you think. That's the problem. You have been ruled since birth by all of the ideas and values from sources outside of yourself. You got stuck in a way of thinking and patterns of behavior that have been handed down from generation to generation. The influence is often gender, cultural and ethnic specific. Add to the mix the familial and community beliefs that we were bombarded with before we were seven years old and had reached the age of reason. By this time we were supposed to know right from wrong. Up until that age, children exist in a Theta brain wave state, which is considered a persistent hypnotic "trance". Using the definition of hypnosis as being in a state of heightened suggestibility, this makes sense.

What all this means is that children come into this world with a clean slate and without preconceived ideas or past experience. Their exposure to different ideas and beliefs is limited because their exploration of anything new or different is limited by virtue of being a child. Therefore, as a child, they have no basis of comparison by which to challenge what they are learning and how they are enculturated. We, as adults, have many layers of ideas, concepts and beliefs about our behavior, our social structure and our moral values or lack thereof as a result of our life experiences. Our global exposure via the news media, the information highway and other forms of instantaneous communication add to the jumble of what we must sort through to learn who we truly are, what we think and how we feel. So, how do you get to be the true you?

Beliefs are crucial to our health, which encompasses the state of our physical, emotional and spiritual WellBeing. Our beliefs are at the crux of how we are *being* now and how we will *be* going forward. As life unfolds, we find ourselves *being* different at various times in our lives. To survive, we change and we adapt what we do. To thrive, we change and adapt what we believe.

In my workshops, I explain positive and negative belief systems in this way. First, remember that we can choose to let go of, disbelieve or replace beliefs that no longer serve our highest good. Think of your belief system as a positively or negatively powered bicycle.

Imagine that you must choose between two bicycles. On one bike, the wheels spin in a negative direction and the wheels of the other bike spin in a positive direction. How can you tell the difference? If you believe that life has handed you lemons, nothing ever goes your way, you feel unworthy and undeserving of the best that life has to offer, than you have chosen the negatively powered bike. If you feel great about yourself, have a totally can-do attitude, have everything that you could ever want or need in life and are doing what brings you joy and contentment, you chose the positively powered bike.

Here is what the negatively powered bike looks like:

NEGATIVE CYCLE OF BEING

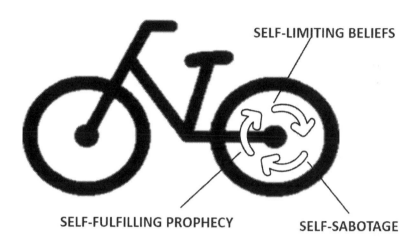

SELF-LIMITING BELIEFS

SELF-FULFILLING PROPHECY

SELF-SABOTAGE

You have inherited a set of beliefs, many of which are self-limiting, and you have compounded them over the years. Any time you try to go beyond those self-limiting beliefs, no matter how badly you want to, you put the brakes on by sabotaging your efforts. Then what happens? You have fulfilled the prophecy of the original negative self-limiting belief, which serves to prove to yourself that you are bound by those negative self-limiting beliefs. *Oy!* Your negatively powered bike can only stand still or roll backwards. Where does that get you? You see, your happiness, WellBeing and joy all hinge on one thing. It's those pesky little self-limiting beliefs. They are fear based, which is felt as that high level of anxiety you experience when the envelope of your comfort zone is pushed or threatened.

Here is what the positively powered bicycle looks like:

POSITIVE CYCLE OF BEING

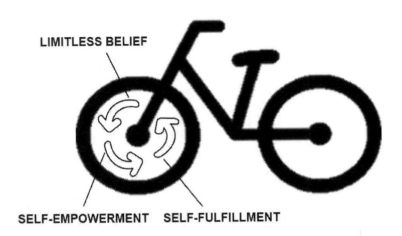

LIMITLESS BELIEF

SELF-EMPOWERMENT SELF-FULFILLMENT

The positively powered bicycle runs on your positive limitless beliefs. You become empowered by raising yourself up to a place of worthiness and deservedness. Achieving self-fulfillment is now possible because you are being who you want to be. *Ah, so much better.*

Having said all that, beliefs are fluid. Some say beliefs are based upon facts. Facts can change as new information comes to light or you as an individual learn or uncover conflicting information. Abraham-Hicks says that a belief is just a thought that you keep thinking. There are many that latch on to a belief or an entire belief system and steadfastly hold on to it despite evidence of its efficacy or of its value to the contrary. Denial or undue influence by others (think cult) plays a huge part as to why beliefs can be so difficult to change or let go. Beliefs keep us in our comfort zone.

I had no idea how many of my beliefs went unquestioned because of my Catholic upbringing and my training as a nurse. There was so much that needed to be challenged, set aside, banished or overridden in finding my path to

WellBeing. I found out that beliefs, truth and facts are all up to interpretation and are subjective according to one's perception. This left me in a state of confusion and a bit of anxiety until I realized that changing my self-limiting beliefs to limitless beliefs gave me 100 percent control over my thoughts and, by extension, my emotions and my physical body.

Some may ask how this is possible, that surely I am indulging in some form of wishful thinking, taking a positive attitude a little too far or that I am delusional. There were many among the healthcare professionals who thought the latter. Some thought that I was just lucky, it was a spontaneous remission or it was, as Barry Manilow says, a "true blue spectacle, a miracle come true". What's true is that my new beliefs, positive attitude and wishful thinking are what allowed me to change how I saw the world and my place in it.

CHAPTER TWENTY

ORDINARY MIRACLES

The Cambridge Dictionary defines a miracle as "an unusual and mysterious event that is thought to have been caused by God as the event does not follow the usual laws of nature". Having been raised Catholic, we were taught that miracles were only bestowed upon a precious few of the most pious, whose fervent prayers were answered by praying to the sainted and the blessed. That made miracles hard to come by. The word miracle comes from *miraculum*, which is Latin for *object of wonder* and certainly broadens the scope of what might be considered ordinary miracles; a sunrise, a child's laughter or even our bodies being designed to self-heal from the tiniest cut on a finger to cancer. These miracles happen every day and yet their origins were created by a higher power. A win-win and everyone goes home happy.

My path to WellBeing was indeed a miracle – an ordinary miracle that I believe we are all capable of achieving and receiving. Upon reflection, there were many miracles big and small along the way that led to the Big Kahuna of Miracles. Some would say it was coincidence, dumb luck, serendipity or synchronicity. I don't believe in coincidences. It has been said that a coincidence is God's way of being anonymous. As for dumb luck, I'm not so dumb and I've never felt that I was particularly lucky. I would say that it was divinely engineered synchronicity. Each event was serendipitously placed in my path that furthered me along on my journey to being healed. All I had to do was recognize the signs, go with my gut and just plain old take a giant leap of faith and grow wings on the way down. That is my definition of a miracle.

Miracles are there for the asking. Just be clear about what you want and then be alert to the signs that your miracle is in the works. We tend to think of miracles as occurring like a bolt out of the blue and randomly hitting someone. I would say that your chances are better to win the Mega Millions lottery than just sitting idly by hoping for a miracle. *Ya gotta be in it to win it!* What I am saying is that you need to be proactive; otherwise, it would be like filling out an employment application and then sleeping with it under your pillow hoping the HR guy will call in the morning and offer you the job.

Miracles aren't always easily recognizable and we don't always get the one we hoped for. I do believe that every prayer is answered and that each soul has its own path to follow despite the wishes of their loved ones. Look around. Be alert and you will discover a miracle where you least expect it. It may not be the big shiny one you asked for, but it's there.

When my cousin Ellen passed a month before I was diagnosed, her family prayed mightily that she would get well. How could she not? Her husband had passed just a year earlier. Her children would be left orphans if she didn't get well. After her death, I encouraged my aunt, uncle and cousins to find the miracles, to keep looking. Isn't it ironic that I was one of those miracles? The miracle for my cousin's family, I believe, is that Ellen and Mike's kids are now thriving and happy. No one would argue that the best case scenario would have been for them to be raised and nurtured by their parents, but things have a way of turning out as they should in the big scheme of things. I know that there are many blessings yet to come for them all of them.

Miracles Come in All Sizes

The many events and sometimes unrecognized miracles go back quite a way. I will list them in chronological order and begin back in April of 2008, which marked the beginning of the cascade of events that ultimately led to my healing.

Miracles #1 and #2

As stated in the Prologue, in April of 2008, I tripped over a little wee stone and tore some ligaments and broke a bone in my right foot.

I developed pain in my right leg and was treated for Achilles tendonitis. One year later, almost to the day I was admitted to the hospital for the same symptoms in my left leg. An ultrasound revealed severe DVTs (blood clots) in my left leg as well as evidence of now-healed blood clots in my right leg.

Okay. So where is the miracle here? The fact that, with one occurrence of misdiagnosed and untreated DVT's in my right leg and the discovery of severe clots in my left leg, I had a total of six major veins affected that badly compromised the circulation to both legs and none of those huge clots broke off and travelled to my heart, my lungs or my brain and killed me.

Miracle #3

I had a follow-up visit with Dr. Cleary in early August and all seemed well. This was Head Cock #1, the first of four head cocks which would signal a major change in my condition. Had Dr. Cleary not ordered the MRA/MRV (special MRI of the arteries and veins) of the pelvis that led to the discovery of the huge tumor, the disease would have continued to spread evermore rapidly and undetected for God knows how long.

Miracle #4

Having Dr. Grace available to take my case was a true blessing. I don't know if I would have had the courage to stand up for myself or to stay strong in the face of another doctor who might not have accepted, respected and supported my beliefs and my intention to be well as Dr. Grace so lovingly did.

Miracle #5

I am including a cluster of those serendipitous synchronicities that fell into my path as I searched for a place to begin my healing sojourn. First was being with my friend, Lois, after the phone call from the hematologist about the MRA/MRV results. Lois had the know-how and the presence of mind to address the fear head-on in those first critical moments. It really set me on my path with greater confidence.

There was that email that had the video from Greg Braden that I inexplicably did not delete. It so strongly influenced me by showing how self-healing was possible. My initial desire to "get rid" of the cancer seemed like a pipe dream. Watching the video over and over made me believe that healing was possible.

The day after the call, I came across a postcard in an ever-growing stack of mail from Abraham-Hicks about their new book called *The Vortex*. I had many of their books and DVDs and did not think that there was anything else I could learn from them. *Silly me*. Besides, I figured I had already given them enough of my money for other books and DVDs, so I tossed it in the trash. That very day, there was another postcard in the mail and I tossed that one too. Then I got an email that evening about the book. *Persistent little buggers*. At first glance, it seemed like the book was mainly about relationships. Who had time for that stuff? I was in a bit of a time crunch here. I was about to delete it when something caught my eye. I don't remember what it was that made me look more closely at the description. It still didn't ring my bell, but I felt an urgency to have this book. The very next day, I went to Barnes and Noble and bought a copy of the book.

As I scanned through it, I was still not getting anything that I would consider useful – at least not then. Later that afternoon, I opened the book to a random page and began to read a passage in the middle of a chapter. I was stunned to read that by applying the Law of Attraction, your body can spontaneously heal. That got my attention. It took a hit upside the head with a two-by-four but it finally got my attention. To paraphrase the passage, even if your body currently hosts every disease known to man, they can all disappear in a moment. There was more to it, of course, but that was the gist of it. I did not quite believe the speed at which they promised complete healing but I had two more weeks left before surgery and I was willing to give it a shot. The book came with a companion audio CD that had that passage. I reread and listened to that section many times a day. I listened to it as I went to sleep at night and I read it first thing every morning. This further emboldened me to pursue complete healing and strengthened my conviction to do my part in making it happen.

Calling upon Roxy for her advice and support felt like it came out of the blue because up until then, our relationship was friendly but collegial. Turns out it was a very good and logical choice. As I said earlier, I felt compelled to call her and I am forever grateful that I did. Her use of hypnosis, Reiki and chakra balancing were comforting and grounding.

Miracle #6

Of course, I must include the bestowing of the *knowing* as a miraculous event. It was the watershed moment in my journey when I heard the words, "It's gone. You're fine," whispered in my ear.

Miracle #7

Who can forget the pedunculated peanut? That polyp in my stomach completely disappeared in less than two weeks and turned out to be the first tangible physical evidence that my body was healing itself.

Miracle #8

Having the interventional radiologist be able to insert the IVC filter through my groin because the tumor was smaller than seen on the previous scan was more proof that things were moving in the right direction.

Miracle #9

The colposcopy showed pristine cervical tissue less than two weeks after a grossly abnormal Pap smear result.

Miracle #10

This was a biggie. Finding no evidence that the cancer had spread anywhere and that the tumor was dying from the inside and was no longer considered to be cancerous was the best news of all. I could finally relax in the knowledge that I was not going to croak due to that nasty disease.

Miracle #11

Some may not consider this a miracle, but my mother's passing allowed her to be there for me in a way that she could never have been even if she were in the best of health in body and mind.

Miracle #12

The "Rhoid Rage" incident turned out to be truly miraculous. I am not being overly dramatic when I say that I could have easily bled to death as evidenced by the need for a transfusion of two units of blood the following day.

Miracle #13

The doctors and nurses were all amazed at how quickly and completely my kidney function returned and the edema (swelling) subsided. What they expected to take weeks, took only a few days.

Miracle #14

Head Cock #2. After getting the go-ahead to be discharged from the hospital after surgery with the plan to take the filter out in a few weeks, the hematologist stopped at the door, cocked her head and decided that I should get the filter removed before I went home. That turned out to be a major blessing given the humongous free-floating blood clot that formed on top of the filter. Once again, I was snatched from the jaws of death.

Miracles #15 and #16

Head Cock #3. As Dr. Grace was walking out the door after my first post-op visit, she stopped at the door and cocked her head and rechecked my incisional site, only to discover the collection of fluid that was inside my surgical wound and, of course, the dreaded tunnel.

Head Cock #4 was the final head cock which came a few weeks later when I developed what was thought to be a mild infection in the tunnel. After prescribing oral antibiotics and about to leave the room, Dr. Grace cocked her head and came back into the room, poked around in the top of the tunnel and opened three huge pockets of pus. Without them being drained, the antibiotics would have been useless in treating the infection. It also would have been very painful and you already know how I feel about pain.

Miracle #17

Beginning with a CA125 (the blood marker for ovarian cancer) of 17,000 and a post-op level of 11 (normal) was astonishing to say the least. The expectation was that it would, hopefully, come down gradually. It was as if the cancer had never been there.

Miracles #18 and #19

In preparing to remove the IVC filters, I had an ultrasound during which time the techs were unable to find any evidence of the huge clot that formed on the top of the IVC filter. That just doesn't happen.

The fact that both filters slipped out like *buttah* without incident after having been in there for five and a half months was amazing even to Dr. Rand, the interventional radiologist. He even called it a miracle as he had never seen one, never mind two, come out so easily after all that time.

I am sure there were other events and instances that could have been considered miraculous. It was just that they were coming so fast and furious, it was hard to keep track. I am so grateful that they all added up to a very happy outcome.

CHAPTER TWENTY-ONE

THE FEAR FACTOR

Having to deal with fear on so many different levels was an ever-present constant on the road to restoring my WellBeing. Fear is a significant and vital part of a cancer diagnosis or even the threat of cancer. I believe that fear is the number one stopper to any forward progress in healing of any kind. It is just that powerful. As I began to prepare for writing this chapter, it occurred to me that in order to make it meaningful, I needed to really break fear down to its core elements. Looking back at each aspect of healing that I have discussed thus far, I noted that they all have been from a retrospective point of view. When this all started, I really didn't know what to do or how to do what I needed to do to be well again. To share with you how I got from there to here, I find that I must reverse engineer the processes that led to my healing. It was important to discuss my spirituality, my beliefs and my many blessings first so that I could lay the groundwork for addressing the subject of fear, which I believe makes it a pivotal chapter in this book. Successfully coping with and yes, banishing fear is the lynch pin upon which hinges the outcome of any disease or obstacle that impedes your WellBeing.

Fear triggers a physiologic response to a real or perceived threat of a physical or an emotional nature. There are three responses to fear. I am sure you are familiar with the first two – the fight or flight response, which is activated when we believe that there is a possibility of outrunning or outfighting an attack. These two responses are about there being some hope of survival. There is a third response in addition to fight or flight, and that is the freeze response. This gets activated when there is no hope of being able to outrun or outfight the threat.

Fight or flight as a response to fear comes with a long list of unpleasant but important physiologic changes necessary to face your foe. The autonomic nervous system causes your pupils to dilate for better vision, your heart rate increases to pump more oxygen into your blood, which gets shunted to your major muscles for greater speed and strength. The sympathetic nervous system triggers the relaxation response when the threat passes. The freeze response causes the body to immobilize. I am sure that you have heard the terms "scared stiff", "frozen with fear" or the "deer in the headlights" (sometimes called the "fawn response"). These are all primitive or *reptilian brain* responses that served us well when saber-toothed tigers roamed the earth.

How does this relate to cancer or any illness that is not immediately life threatening? When I received the phone call from the hematologist to tell me that there was a huge mass in my pelvis and knowing that the odds were overwhelmingly indicative of ovarian cancer, I felt the threat to my mortal self. I suppose I could have dropped the phone and run away (flight). I could have smashed the phone as it was the instrument that delivered the threat (fight). My response was to freeze. Cancer had become my saber-toothed tiger. I could not outrun it or outfight it. My only option was to play dead. I became immobilized. I shut down. I dissociated from the reality of it. This was not a choice. It

was the only survival mechanism at my dispos
moment.

I could have become stuck in this state. U
or flight response where the energy is diss..
sympathetic nervous system when the threat passes, energy
from the freeze response can be pent up, as there may be no
awareness of ever experiencing the freeze response and its
consequences. This means that shutting down closes off
much of the trauma of the incident. Having dealt with many
patients and clients facing similar situations, I recognized
that despite being in shock, I needed to find a way to move
forward. The only way to do this was to deal with the fear. I
have said before that I was able to rather quickly move past
the initial "attack", although I don't believe that I fully
released the "stuck" energy.

Recognizing the fear in all of its forms as more and more
of the reality of my situation sank in was challenging indeed.
As I said, the freeze response was not a choice. How I
handled what came next was a choice, however. Running
away from it all was never an option for me. Giving in to the
hype and hoopla around cancer was not particularly
appealing to me either. I chose to be well. I chose not to
think of myself as sick. I chose not to focus on the disease. I
chose not to fight cancer. I chose to focus on reclaiming my
WellBeing. Note, I said WellBeing, not getting well. If I am
not thinking of my state of WellBeing, then I am thinking of
my lack of wellness. It may sound like semantics to you,
however, the difference between the two is huge to me. I
kept my eye on the prize at all times.

How was I able to make those choices? I did it by
keeping the fear at bay. But how? The choices I made did not
allow room for the fear to override my desire for WellBeing.
In essence, I really didn't *do* anything about the fear. It went
away when my thoughts, beliefs and actions left no room for
it to rear its ugly head. Remember when you were younger

d there was always one kid who was an itch? Someone would invariably say to ignore him and he'll go away. He didn't always go away but when you stopped feeding his need for attention by responding to him, he stopped being an itch, or at least you stopped noticing him.

Along my journey, I encountered many more challenges or setbacks and the fear would come roaring back. As time went by, the roar became weaker and weaker. I no longer felt that fear was the enemy. It was not something that I needed to beat back, conquer or battle. It was a physiologic response that I could handle and release when my threat assessment for things beyond my control allowed for more reasonable and rational options. For example, I thought better feeling thoughts. You cannot hold two thoughts of conflicting or contrasting emotional impact at the same time, so I just chose the better feeling one.

WARNING: Wallowing in fear is hazardous to your health!

I know this sounds too simple to be that easy. It *is* simple but I never said it was easy. It takes practice but it is doable. Practice it even when your threat alert level is low. Just practice thinking thoughts that are better feeling than the ones that make you feel mad or bad or sad.

I am not suggesting that you ignore fearful feelings or situations altogether. In the process of healing (yes, my body had to heal and it healed because I focused on my WellBeing), I encountered many situations and received information that was fear provoking. I recognized the fear for what it was. Fear is an early warning threat alert system that allows you to prepare for a comfortable and safe way to handle fearful situations or events. I did not always get a grip on fear attacks in a timely manner and I accumulated more than my share of stuck energy over time. Because it went unrecognized and untreated, I suffered from PTSD.

Fortunately for me, my therapist, Doris, recognized the signs early on and we worked through it.

The best thing that I would recommend to anyone facing a life crisis is to get some help from supportive family, friends, a mental health professional, a health coach or an energy healing practitioner; preferably, all of the above. Set aside your embarrassment or shame and do it. It is all part of reclaiming and maintaining your WellBeing.

My coach, Evie M. Caprel, shares her story of how fear can escalate because of preprogrammed beliefs.

It was a day like any other. Except my mom died that day. The day before my twelfth birthday.

June 10, 1969. Ten years earlier, she had been diagnosed with breast cancer. She already had a mastectomy and I later learned the disease had spread to her bones. Death was inevitable back then. Fast forward to decades later. I had my first mammogram at age thirty-one. I also went through years of therapy in my forties to understand and cope with the trauma of losing a mother as a young child. I thought that I learned to deal with the fear of the disease by staying healthy, eating well, being physically active, and nurturing myself, my husband and my family...everything "they" tell you to do to stay healthy.

Let me state right now: I am completely healthy. Although every once in a while, the fear of the disease insidiously creeps into my mind. Recently, when I got out of bed in the morning, I experienced a sharp pain in my left breast, but then it would dissipate within a few seconds. I didn't think much of it, but after it continued for a few weeks, my curiosity and anxiety began to mount. I am a strong proponent of integrative healthcare and contacted my most trusted alternative health professional.

He asked, "Where is the pain?" Okay, I was starting to get scared. The fear was mounting. The little voice in my head starting pitching lightning bolts of doubt in my mind as I waited for his reply. "After all I've done to stay healthy." "What is happening?" "I don't want to go into 'that world'."

The Fear-o-Meter was in the red. Ready to explode. It's nearly impossible to be present with anyone or anything when the fear takes over. Then I remembered a passage from an article that Pat had written about how she had worked through her fear. I started my deep breathing.

I imagined my breasts healthy and happy. I repeated, "I am healthy. All is well." The fear subsided. A calm understanding blanketed me: my mother's health journey is not my fate. I love and miss her, but I do not have to take on her experience.

"I am healthy. All is well." Pat's "Healing Triad" brought me smoothly back to releasing the fear and focusing on the path to WellBeing again. A much more powerful way to be.

I have often heard the acronym for fear is **F**alse **E**vidence **A**ppearing **R**eal. Sometimes the evidence is real and there is a real reason for concern. The goal is to deal with the fear so that appropriate and productive action can be taken. On a lighter note, I offer several humorous acronyms for fear that may suit your situation:

F**k **E**verything **A**nd **R**esist (Fight)
F**k **E**verything **A**nd **R**etreat (Flight)
F**k **E**verything **A**nd **R**est (Freeze)

CHAPTER TWENTY-TWO

ENERGY IS ALL THAT MATTERS

No story of healing would be complete without a little something about energy; the origin of everything. You don't have to be a quantum physicist to grasp the concept of energy being at the crux of all that is. Not so long ago, I scoffed at the new age woo-wooers who claimed to be "energy workers" and could facilitate healing by delivering, manipulating or raising the vibration of energy. I can now appreciate and understand that all matter is energy and energy is all that really matters. Still the depth of my knowledge regarding energy would scarcely fill a thimble from the vastness of our infinite universe.

In the most general terms, energy has many forms including kinetic, potential, electromagnetic and nuclear, to name a few. I feel compelled to add spiritual and emotional energy to that list. Energy causes things to happen or change. It can move or transform objects and it can be transferred from one object to another. Energy can neither be created nor destroyed. What was once thought to be emptiness or dead space between the tiniest of subatomic particles, we now know is pure energy. It is known as the matrix or the unified field that exists around and between all of that which has mass.

A recently identified subatomic element called the Higgs boson theoretically acts like a glue that gives all matter mass. It has been dubbed the *God Particle*. Could this answer the question as to how God can be everywhere? Just considering that this is an answerable question puts a limit on the limitless nature of an infinite God and therefore remains unanswerable. It would be easier to lasso a waterfall.

One might wonder what any of this has to do with healing. It has everything to do with healing. Energy is not just about holding physical mass together. It is about the confluence of our thoughts, beliefs and physiology, at a cellular level, that allows healing to take place and for WellBeing to prevail.

This is not just new age fluff. There is science to back this stuff up. Dr. Bruce Lipton is a cellular biologist and pioneer in stem cell research. Through his work in the revolutionary field of behavioral epigenetics, Dr. Lipton found that environment, thoughts, perceptions, and beliefs can affect genes. This means that we are not held hostage by nor must we fall victim to our genetic makeup. In his book, *The Biology of Belief*, he says, "Thoughts have a profound [*positive*] effect on behavior and genes but *only* when they are in harmony with subconscious programming [*our belief system*]...negative thoughts have an equally powerful effect." Quite simply, your emotions, created by thought, regulate your genetic expression. Dr. Lipton further states that up until recently, "...conventional researchers have completely ignored the role that energy plays in health and disease." Claiming control of my WellBeing and taking action to radically retool my beliefs, thoughts and emotions, I was able to experience, first-hand, the role energy played in my own extraordinary healing.

For the energetically uninitiated, these are a few terms that are bandied about when speaking of energy healing. The first and most frequently used is vibration, which is defined as a back and forth movement or oscillation. All energy has a vibration including animate and inanimate objects as well as thoughts and emotions. Information is carried by vibration. Remember the saying about computer programming? Garbage in, garbage out. It is the same with our bodies. Let's use food as an example. Crappy food delivers crappy information to the body just as high quality food delivers high quality information.

Frequency reflects the number of vibratory oscillations per second representing one cycle called a hertz. My father was a civil engineer and I heard him talk about this stuff all the time, but I always thought it was only about electricity. Now I understand that we are all frequency generators. The faster the emotional vibration, the higher the frequency. In terms of our health, that's a good thing. Conversely, slower means lower and that's a bad thing.

The last term is vibrational frequency and it is often used interchangeably with vibration. Thought is the most potent energy form there is because it has no boundaries or limitations. We create our thoughts based on our belief system. Thoughts create vibration. The vibration of our thoughts creates emotions which pass the information along to our physical bodies. Changing our beliefs consequently changes our thoughts giving us control over our vibrational frequency and ultimately control over our physical and emotional health. *Simple, right?*

Just as illness begins with a thought, so too does healing. Choose your thoughts consciously and carefully and you choose WellBeing by default. Our bodies seek equilibrium. Creating a state of harmonious resonance allows us to achieve balance. But how? By raising our vibration. This might be easier to grasp by considering what Abraham-

ys about the Emotional Scale in the book (which I highly recommend), *Ask and It is Given*. There is a hierarchy of emotions ranging from the depth of despair to the height of joyfulness and every other emotion in between. Think of emotions as being in Red, Yellow or Green Zones. Fear, for example, is way down near the bottom of the Red Zone and vibrates at a very low frequency which can create a state of inertia. Joy, which is at the very top of the Green Zone, would be preferable with its high vibrational frequency. Getting from the Red Zone all the way up to the Green Zone all at once would require a giant leap.

Raising your vibration is easiest to achieve, gradually, by reaching for a better feeling thought. This may seem a little odd but anger, worry and doubt are an improvement over fear, albeit they are still in the Red Zone. Moving into overwhelm, frustration and impatience is not optimal yet it gets you out of the Red Zone and into the Yellow Zone, allowing you to better take positive action on your own behalf. When you are able to feel, even fleetingly, hopefulness, positive expectation or optimism, you have reached the Green Zone and this is cause for celebration. The vibrational frequency of emotions in the Green Zone is where healing takes place.

A little side note:
Coming out.

In the early '90s, when I first began to embrace the concepts of energy and vibration, I stayed as far back in the woo-woo closet as I possibly could for fear that I would be seen as a card-carrying member of the lunatic fringe.

One evening while having dinner with a group of friends, I outed myself and have never regretted it for a moment. There was a woman, whom I did not know well, complaining about her bitter divorce and how she would lose everything (money and material possessions). She asked (jokingly, I thought) of the few of us who were nurses if there was a way that she could kill her husband and not leave a trace of evidence. While that was not part of our curriculum in nursing school, we engaged in some hypothetical speculation to humor her. Our light-hearted approach did nothing to assuage her rage and her vitriolic diatribe continued well past appetizers and into the main course. No amount of cajoling or attempts to change the subject could sway her focus.

I was becoming uncomfortable, as were all of the other guests. The heaviness of our collective mood was palpable as we all felt the energy being sucked out of the room. She was, single-handedly, lowering the vibrational frequency of nine other people. It was not long before everyone else took up the mantle and began to bitch and moan about significant others in their lives. It seemed that anybody not present was fair game. I wondered if anything could salvage what had begun as a nice evening with friends.

I felt as if I was on a runaway train with no way to stop it. I did not want to risk having this angry mob turn on me for being a Pollyanna but my anxiety was mounting and I needed to do something positive. When one friend was ragging on a coworker, whom we all knew and liked, I made my move. I said that although he was not perfect as few of us are, we had to admit that he had a kind heart and a beautiful soul. Then I listed a few of his more flattering attributes to back up my claim. After a moment of awkward silence, several people began to agree that he did indeed have many redeeming qualities. With a little more prodding, the conversation took a pleasant turn. By dessert, we all came up with a few nice things to say about each other and to proclaim that each of us had a kind heart and a beautiful soul.

At the end of the evening, we were all able to raise our vibrational frequency from the Red Zone all the way up *into the Green Zone...well, except for the bitter soon-to-be divorcée, who was only able to move up into the Yellow Zone – but hey, it was a start.*

It may seem as if I have gone far afield of my initial discussion about energy, however, I believe that I have come full circle because no healing would be possible without the presence of energy. This was not an easy concept for me to wrap my head around and I, by no means, have all the answers. Energy is a subject that is far too vast to adequately cover here in this book or in a thousand other books. My inner healer is okay about not having all the answers. The nurse in me is not okay with that. My inner two year old, however, keeps them both satisfied by incessantly asking, "Why?" content in knowing that the answers we seek will eventually be revealed.

I have made no bones about being more spiritual than religious. Having said that, the Bible has much to offer by way of explaining the unexplainable. For example, in Colossians 1:16 can be found this passage:

"For by Him were all things created, that are in heaven, and that are in earth, visible and invisible, whether [they be] thrones, or dominions, or principalities, or powers: all things were created by Him, and through Him. And He is before all things..."

There is more that is unknown about healing and energy than is known. While science tries to figure it all out, it is our faith in a higher power that allows us to heal without having to know how or why. We need only believe that we can.

CHAPTER TWENTY-THREE

SELFIES

Radical Self-Care

Healing an illness is a good thing. Doing it with no or minimal traditional medical intervention is an even better thing. Not getting sick is the best thing of all.

This book has focused mainly on my own self-healing from a devastating and life-threatening disease. I pulled out all the stops and brought out the big metaphysical and spiritual guns, aiming them, metaphorically speaking, at the cancer. I was very pleased with myself for accomplishing this healing and rested on my laurels for quite some time. I just whipped out my belief change bazooka and *poof*, the cancer was gone. *Well, not quite like that.*

I thought that I was bulletproof. No disease or condition was a match for my secret weapon. Then I realized that I had spent all of my energy and focus on healing one disease. Yes, the cancer was gone, however, I still had a laundry list of age-related, stress-related and neglect-related issues that had manifested in my physical body. I had accommodated them all without much notice over the years. I was too busy as a nurse trying to save the rest of the world from disease and pestilence.

I had ignored the most basic tenet of my nurse's training; that is, caring for all aspects of a patient as a fully integrated individual from a holistic point of view. I had never considered the impact that the denial of self-care was taking on me as a physical, emotional and spiritual being. I recognized the ramifications of that denial from my patients and yet, I never held a mirror up to my own shortcomings. Self-care is at the very heart of a nurse's obligation to be of service to the sick. This is, actually, true for any caregiver.

So what is self-care, exactly? The World Health Organization defines self-care as "activities individuals, families, and communities undertake with the intention of enhancing health, preventing disease, limiting illness, and restoring health." The American Holistic Nurses Association states that the principle of self-care is a critical component of nursing. Nurses must recognize that they cannot facilitate healing unless they are in the process of healing themselves.

On the surface, self-care means taking care of yourself, but I'm sure you figured that out on your own. On a much deeper level, self-care does not come so easily for most of us. Many of us are givers by nature or necessity, always putting the needs of others first. We do this because of the multiple roles we play that require a selfless devotion to a job, parenthood, caring for sick or elderly parents or a spouse. We do it out of a sense of love, obligation, duty, guilt or even martyrdom.

The real question is, who takes care of you? The answer I hear most often is "nobody". This is where everyone gets stuck because being a caregiver leaves you no time for you. Someone else always needs you more, or maybe you don't think you deserve to be cared for. Here is a simple truth. If no one else is stepping up to the plate for you, then you need to step up for yourself. I am willing to bet, however, that you do get offers of help and cast them aside or they go unnoticed because you are unaccustomed to caring for yourself in a loving way. A prescription for self-care requires a hefty dose of self-love. This is easier said than done and requires a bit (a lot in my case) of practice. Think about this. The airlines got one thing absolutely correct. The safety procedures call for a parent to put their own oxygen mask on first in case of an emergency before assisting their child. If you are unable to breathe, you cannot help anyone else. So, for the chronic caregiver, self-care allows you to have more strength and stamina to be of service to others. If you're not sure if you are a chronic caregiver, ask yourself these questions:

Are you reluctant to ask for help?
Do you have difficulty accepting help?
Are you always the last item on your To Do List?
Do you even make it onto your To Do List?
Are you a Wounded Healer? That is someone who desperately needs the care and attention that they so selflessly give to others but never allows the time for themselves to receive or accept it.

If you answered yes to any of the above questions, the likelihood of you being a chronic caregiver is quite high.

During the past five years, this was not a lesson that I learned easily or quickly, despite all that I had been through. It honestly never occurred to me that I could or should apply the same self-healing tools I learned while healing the cancer to the other health issues. *I never claimed to be the sharpest knife in the drawer.* Not long ago, during a week-long respite of quiet contemplation on a beautiful beach in southern Florida, it came to me that I had gotten my free pass with the cancer and I was going to have to do the work for the rest of my healing. I needed to fully and radically

se long-forgotten tenets of self-care. But how? I
lowing these five basic tenets of self-care:

nore of what you love and less of what you don't
love.

2. Embrace the 80/20 Principle which, in the most simple terms, means letting go of the 80 percent of the joyless crap in your life and focus on the joyful 20 percent.

3. Figure out what feeds your mind, body and spirit.

4. Commit to "indulge" yourself regularly. Don't just pencil it in. Make it sacrosanct.

5. Watch your language. This means cutting out the negative self-talk and the stinkin' thinkin' and replace it with empowering and loving thoughts and words.

Self-care is selfish and that's okay.

This quote from Abraham-Hicks sums it all up for me. "Entertaining yourself, pleasing yourself, connecting with yourself, being yourself, enjoying yourself, loving yourself. Some say, 'Well, Abraham you teach selfishness.' And we say, yes we do, yes we do, yes we do, because unless you are selfish enough to reach for that connection, you don't have anything to give anyone, anyway. And when you are selfish enough to make that connection – you have an enormous gift that you give everywhere you are."

Radical Self-Care means committing to a self-determined regimen of scheduled activities as well as adopting a way of being that encompasses the above Five Tenets of Self-Care. What's radical about that? The fact that self-care is an alien concept to the chronic caregiver makes embracing those self-care tenets a radical departure from the occasional assortment of half-hearted attempts to "take a break".

Self-Directed Healing

I have shared my story from an illness/healing point of view and I hope that it has inspired you to seek your own healing from a place of strength and empowerment. I encourage you to leave your past health missteps behind you today and move forward from a place of confidence and belief in yourself as you begin your own healing journey. Later, I will share in greater detail the techniques, tools and tips that I used in my own healing that I have found to be of benefit along my ongoing WellBeing journey.

I am not offering my path to WellBeing as a blueprint for all to follow. I was guided along this path as you will be guided along yours when you are open to receiving it without resistance.

It is often said that there is not much to be gained by closing the barn door after the horses get out. There is also no use in crying over spilled milk. The past is water under the bridge or over the dam. These are but a few of the American colloquialisms we are so fond of uttering when life does not unfold as planned. I am sure there are plenty more like these in every language. Is this all empty rhetoric or might it be helpful to glean some value from this perspective? The takeaway here is to move forward and not beat yourself up about the past.

Self-directed healing assumes that something needs to be healed. After the cancer, there remained several other health issues that were vying for the top spot. I continue to be a work in progress. After all, Rome wasn't built in a day.

Self-Directed WellBeing

These days, I allow myself to choose the what, who, how and where of my wellness. I decided it is better to close the barn door *before* the horses get out. I needed to take control of my wellness, which I now call Self-Directed WellBeing. This simply means that I choose to focus on being well and staying well, which required another shift in my thinking and believing. This is really a pivotal shift in my mindset, as it impacts my own sense of WellBeing and how I interact with the healthcare establishment. This is a radical departure from how we as a society view healthcare.

Soap Box Alert!

Let me just point out that the delivery of healthcare offers very little in terms of supporting your health. What we have is a disease management system. We wait until we are sick to access healthcare. What's wrong with this picture? Insurance companies pay for cancer hunts under the guise of health screenings for breast, colon, cervical and prostate cancer, to name a few, but they don't pay much mind to wellness maintenance. They give lip service to prevention but what they are really selling is early detection wrapped up to look like prevention.

The idea that I could direct my own healing and wellness through the integration of conventional medicine, CAM and behavioral epigenetics is an extremely freeing feeling. To invoke the nautical metaphor once again, I am now the captain of my own ship. I have recruited a navigator (sometimes more than one) and a crew. My navigator, at any given time, may be a primary care physician with an open mind, a nurse, health coach or naturopath, for example. My crew ebbs and flows as needed and may be comprised of any number of CAM practitioners, from an Acupuncturist to a Zen master and anything and everything in between. To this roster I would also add spiritual advisor, clergy as needed or desired along with supportive friends and family members.

During my WellBeing restoration voyage, I had, inadvertently, assembled my crew, a very large crew indeed. There were, of course, the many medical specialists led by Dr. Grace, my personal cheering squad and my friends and colleagues in the alternative healing arts. I initially referred to them as my Healing Team. I now refer to them as my WellBeing Team. I was, at the time, unaware of just how much control of my WellBeing I had taken. It was, clearly, not evident to the traditionalists, who thought they were still in charge. I had no interest in a power struggle. I didn't need to be right; I just needed to be well.

CHAPTER TWENTY-FOUR

MAY I HAVE YOUR INTENTION PLEASE?

W riting this book has been a real eye-opener for me. At the time of the diagnosis, I felt ill-prepared and ill-equipped to handle the seemingly insurmountable task of complete healing. Looking back, I can now see that I had unknowingly spent the previous fifteen years preparing for that occasion. Why?

It strikes me as kind of funny that as I shared my experience early on, the process seemed to have been quite methodical and well thought out. On the surface, nothing could be further from the truth. Each day I struggled with the fear and doubt, and each day a little bit more of my path was revealed to me. It was as if the path would take a twist or turn just as I felt I was getting my bearings. Perhaps seeing the entire landscape would have been too overwhelming for me. One thing was very clear to me, however – my goal was to come through this adventure well and whole. Indeed, I would be even better than before.

What I never really gave much thought to was that I very emphatically set my intention to be healed, to be completely well...no half measures. It was a winner-take-all proposition. I was not interested in hoping they got all of the cancer or

ot spread as far as they feared. I never saw
g chemo or radiation or being sick in any way. It
ot on my radar.

ot until recently that I began to give the whole
idea of intention some serious thought and consideration. I
was aware that I set a very clear intention to be well,
however, I never really gave the importance of deliberately
setting my intention its due until now. I remember, as part
of my spiritual sojourn, I bought every book by every
modern-day spiritual guru that someone further along their
path would recommend. I bought Wayne Dyer's book, *The
Power of Intention* in 2004 and I absolutely could not get
through the first chapter. I just didn't get it and so I put it
aside. Over the next few years, I had followed the teachings
of a few others including Abraham-Hicks, Deepak Chopra,
Andrew Weil and others. Somewhere along the way, this
stuff started to click. I unearthed Dr. Dyer's book a few years
later and was blown away by the wisdom and simplicity of
his words and ideas. *Timing is everything*. Dr. Dyer is
quoted as saying, "Change the way you look at things and the
things you look at change."

There is great profundity in this statement and there is
also scientific evidence to back it up. Another book that I
had set aside as too deep was *The Intention Experiment* by
Lynne McTaggart from 2007. I gave this book another look-
see after I began to ponder the idea of intention and healing.
Once again, I was amazed at the power of our consciousness
to effect change in ourselves and in the world. Intention can
be defined as a purposeful plan of action leading to a desired
outcome. A desire simply means focusing on the outcome
without any particular plan or strategy in mind to achieve
results.

Facing a life-threatening illness provokes a deep desire
to be well and activates the survival mode in all of us. While
a desire may be strong, it requires no real strategy. Jacking

up that desire by kicking the survival mode into high gear with a strong intention for a clear vision of the outcome makes all the difference in the world. Setting an intention requires commitment, purpose and a plan of action for a very specific result.

It is all too easy to forget about intention as a means of getting what we want and need from life. Remember *The Secret*? It was a movie and a book that urged one and all to invoke the Law of Attraction to get an endless abundance of wealth, health and love just by focusing on what you want. It had some good ideas, however, it left you standing in the doorway of desire with no clear intention. Marilyn Schlitz of the Institute of Noetic Sciences defines intention as "projecting of the awareness, with purpose and efficacy, toward some object or outcome...to influence physical matter...thought had to be highly motivated and targeted."

I ultimately did come up with a plan, although somewhat on the fly. My intention was always focused and I continued moving toward my goal of being well. I was very clear on what I wanted and equally as clear about what I did not want. That is the key if we are to believe in the Law of Attraction (which I do), so it makes sense to focus on what you want.

I said way back in the beginning about not worrying about the cursed "hows". I did leave the *how* everything was going to happen up to the Universe and focused on exactly what I wanted as an outcome. I wanted the cancer gone without the need for chemo and radiation. In the beginning, I was trying to envision how my body would make it all go away. I pictured the tumor melting. Then I thought about where that gooey mess would go and it was just too gross to think about. Truthfully, I really didn't care if it popped out of my belly button as long as it was gone.

All of the steps along the way, from quelling my fears to healing my body by radically changing my beliefs and healing with focused intention, did not happen in a vacuum. My entire experience showed me the irrefutable proof that we truly are all One.

Prior to this, I believe that I, as so many of us do, suffered from IDD or Intention Deficit Disorder. I try (even though trying implies the possibility of failure) to make intention setting as part of my daily routine. It works for the little stuff as well as the big stuff. It just takes a little practice...and patience.

CHAPTER TWENTY-FIVE

NO RIBBONS 'ROUND
MY OLD OAK TREE

At the risk of offending some, I must admit that I am not a big fan of those disease-of-the-month ribbons. It had gotten to the point where I refused to wear pink. I like pink. I look good in pink, however, I do not want to think about breast cancer when I wear pink or when I see those ubiquitous pink ribbons, especially in October, and I really love the month of October. September is the month for ovarian cancer awareness. I like September too. Teal is the color for ovarian cancer awareness. I really like teal and I really look good in teal. Soon, I will be running out of colors I can wear without being reminded of some type of cancer. Now, I am all for the idea of awareness, however, I prefer my reminders for awareness to be of WellBeing and not ones that scare the crap out of me.

I was having lunch with a friend in early October, just a few weeks after getting out of the hospital. In fact, it was my first social outing. We went to a well-known franchise restaurant that was replete with pink ribbons. They were on the coasters, the napkins and there was even a special pink dessert and pink drink on the menu. There were pink ribbons everywhere with the names of patrons who had donated a dollar or two for the cause. I was beginning to lose my appetite.

It was difficult for me to enjoy my lunch with the constant visual barrage of cancer reminders. The last thing I wanted to do right then or ever, for that matter, was to think about cancer. Certainly not in the fearful way it is presented by the media, the healthcare industry, big pharma and the myriad of ribbon campaigns. They are all fear based. It is as if cancer is lurking around every corner, lying in wait for you to miss your Pap smear or mammogram. It is not just cancer. It is heart disease, diabetes, restless leg syndrome, etc. You name it; they'll find a way to make it scary.

My intention is not to knock the good that has come from the pink ribbon campaign or any organization with a desire to help people restore or maintain their health. I just think the message being delivered needs some tweaking.

Remember the fight, flight or freeze responses? Living things, from humans all the way down to the tiniest single-celled organism, move away from pain (fear) and gravitate toward pleasure (WellBeing). I believe these fear tactics may be backfiring in terms of improving early detection with cancer screenings. The messages evoking fear can cause the flight or freeze alarms to sound. These fear-based tactics in advertising, healthcare promotion and with the media sensationalizing it all has got to stop. It is the wrong message and the negativity around the doom and gloom approach is harmful to maintaining a sense of WellBeing.

How is it harmful? How often does someone seek medical help only when symptoms become so severe or a disease is too far advanced? Very often. I can attest to that from my personal and nursing experience. Partly to blame is the limited or nonexistent access to medical care for some, however, the most frequently heard answer is that people are afraid. Yes it is denial; the ignore-it-and-it-will-go-away approach.

If people were not so afraid that every lump, bump and pain was a terminal disease, they might get help earlier. Cancer is so often the first thing that springs to mind. The truth is, it's not always cancer and cancer is not always a death sentence.

It occurred to me that instead of designating days, weeks or months to draw awareness to some dreaded disease, why not celebrate awareness of our WellBeing every single day? In my world, cancer screenings would be called Wellness Screenings. Cancer centers would be called Wellness Centers and cancer treatment would be called Wellness Restoration Care.

The cover of this book depicts the caduceus emerging from the lotus blossom which blooms clean and fragrant, rising above the muddy water in which it is rooted. It embodies purity, enlightenment and faith. The caduceus has evolved to represent the emblem of modern medicine. Together, the marriage of these two symbols, that I call the "*Loduceus*" (pronounced *low-due-sus*) signify healing and WellBeing of the Mind, Body and Spirit.

It is my hope that the *Loduceus* will offer an alternative to those who would prefer awareness of health and Wellbeing, rather than the multi-colored myriad of disease-of-the-month ribbons that harken fearful awareness.

If there are those who still think that some body parts need their own colored ribbon, then at least the message should be to remind us of, for example, beautiful healthy breasts when you see the color pink. How hard could that be? Men do this all the time without any color to remind them.

Off my soapbox and back to lunch.

CHAPTER TWENTY-SIX

TECHNIQUES

Techniques

Following is an overview of the techniques that I employed during my healing journey and how each was of benefit for me personally. They are in no particular order of chronology or importance. I credit them all for their role in calming me, quelling my fears, helping me remain true to my authentic self, radically overhauling my belief system and for my complete physical, emotional and spiritual healing.

I would encourage anyone to seek out these and other integrative modalities, as there is no one-size-fits-all approach to healing. Trying out several modalities even if you are not in any kind of crisis mode can be helpful and enjoyable for your general WellBeing. With my background as a practitioner of several modalities and knowing many wonderful practitioners, I had been able to experience many different techniques over the years. I chose the ones that resonated the most with me for my healing.

Check Recommendations and Resources for a listing of other beneficial techniques and specific tools that may be helpful to you.

PSYCH-K

PSYCH-K is a set of principles and processes designed to change subconscious beliefs that limit the expression of your full potential as a spiritual being having a human experience according to its originator, Rob Williams.

It is a non-invasive, interactive process that is both simple and powerful. PSYCH-K is designed to change subconscious beliefs that are self-limiting and self-sabotaging to beliefs that are unlimited and self-empowering. It was developed by incorporating a unique blend of various tools for change, from ancient mind/body wisdom to contemporary neuroscience research that are effective in the areas of behavioral/habit change, wellness and stress reduction.

Upon hearing about the presence of that big honkin' tumor, my first thought was that it was cancer (a belief based on an educated assumption) and that it would kill me (a severely self-limiting and self-sabotaging belief). This was the very first modality that I used to begin the belief change process. My friend, Lois, and I had taken the PSYCH-K Basic and Advanced courses the year before and, quite honestly, this was the first time either of us had used it. We got out the cheat sheets and got down to business. Within minutes, I was able to begin to settle my fears and believe that I would be well. I believe that this set the course for my ultimately successful healing. PSYCH-K was ground zero and I have since incorporated this easy and effective technique into my practice.

Emotional Freedom Techniques

Emotional Freedom Techniques, better known as EFT or "Tapping", is an energy mobilizing technique that encompasses several aspects of acupuncture, neuro-linguistic programming (NLP), energy medicine/psychology, and Thought Field Therapy (TFT). According to Gary Craig, the founder of EFT, "it is a universal healing tool that can provide impressive results for physical, emotional, and performance issues. EFT operates on the premise that no matter what part of your life needs improvement, there are unresolved emotional issues in the way. Even for physical issues, chronic pain, or diagnosed conditions, it is common knowledge that any kind of emotional stress can impede the natural healing potential of the human body."

In a nutshell, one taps gently with the fingertips on various meridian or acupressure points of the hands, face, head and chest while focusing in on an emotional or physical issue. The idea behind EFT is that all negative emotions are caused by a disruption in the body's energy system. Focusing on the issue will re-establish the flow of energy, thereby releasing the unpleasant feelings. This is an over-simplification of EFT and I would urge everyone to learn more about it.

I have been a practitioner of EFT since 1996 and have been teaching this technique to nurses, moms, dads, kids and really just about anyone who will sit still long enough to let me. It is easy to learn and simple to master the rudiments for your own personal use.

EFT is a technique that I relied heavily upon throughout my healing odyssey. Initially I used it to help quell my fears and calm my nerves. I am a huge fan of tapping because of its effectiveness, its versatility and the convenience it affords the tapper. It is gaining wide acceptance in mainstream medicine. It was recently featured on Dr. Oz and given his stamp of approval.

Switchwords

In his book, *The Secret of Perfect Living,* James T. Mangan created a system that encouraged one to engage the subconscious mind to obtain specific mental states by focusing their attention on mantra-like one-word affirmations called Switchwords. You have already seen how powerful a single word can be. Merely seeing the word cancer in print, hearing it spoken or simply thinking of the word causes an emotional and often physical response. It may be mild or gut-wrenching, but that word does get a reaction from just about everybody. Switchwords are always used in a positive way for positive results. For example, repeating the word WOMB evokes a sense of safety. REACH helps one to find a lost object, a solution to a problem or to recall a forgotten thought or idea.

I had been dabbling with Switchwords for years just for fun. I dusted them off when I needed to gather everything at my disposal for my tool belt. I opted to use what are called Switchphrases which are several Switchwords strung together to potentiate the power of each word for a single goal. The words I chose were designed to help rid myself of the "crabs" once and for all. My Switchphrase for complete healing was DIVINE-ZERO-BE-EXTINCT-TOGETHER. The reason I chose these words will be obvious to you. DIVINE means to work miracles. ZERO means gone; all dried up. BE means to be at peace and in good health. EXTINCT means no longer in existence and TOGETHER is the Mac Daddy of all Switchwords. It means to be single-minded of purpose; to be all as one in harmony.

You can say your words or phrases out loud, you can sing them, chant them or just plain old think them to yourself. I decided to sing mine. The song I chose was "Joy to the World" – the Christmas one, not Three Dog Night. Although that could work too. Try it but I warn you that you will never be able to get the tune out of your head.

Not wanting to alarm the hospital staff by singing a Christmas song in September with seemingly random and bizarre lyrics, I opted to repeat the phrase silently over and over as I did my EFT tapping. It was at that very moment that I was blessed with the *knowing*. I'm pretty sure that was no coincidence. My mind and body were in a state of calm receptivity and it was awesome.

Reiki

Reiki is a technique for stress reduction, relaxation and physical, emotional and spiritual healing. Founded by Mikao Usui in Japan, the word *Reiki* means "spiritually guided life force energy." Administered by placing the hands on the body or just hovering above it, life force energy or Qi (pronounced *chee*) flows through the practitioner allowing the recipient to experience calm, peace, serenity and healing on many levels. It is very effective by itself and may be integrated with more traditional allopathic treatments or other modalities from the alternative healing arts.

Reiki is a simple, natural and safe technique that anyone can use and is taught in three levels. Level I Reiki is, specifically, to allow individuals to use it for their own personal self-improvement and self-healing.

This was one of the first modalities that I sought out because my head was spinning like a top from the overload of emotions and information I was trying to sort out and cope with. Reiki is often the go-to modality that I seek out to this day when I am feeling overwhelmed by stuff when life gets too hectic or I need to make a big decision.

Mikao Usui used the following mantra as a daily meditation. Whether you are a Reiki practitioner or not, these are some powerful ideals to embrace.

Reiki Mantra
Just for today, I will let go of anger
Just for today, I will let go of worry
Just for today, I will give thanks for many blessings
Just for today, I will do my work honestly
Just for today, I will be kind to my neighbor and every living thing

Hypnosis

Habits, like rules, are meant to be broken when they no longer serve a purpose. For my purpose, changing beliefs was the habit I wanted to break. Beliefs are formed at the unconscious level. Why at the unconscious level? Well, beliefs take root in the unconscious mind where the repetitive thoughts become our truth because the unconscious mind accepts, as fact, all information it is given whether it is actually true or not, whether it is actually good for you or not. It follows that since these patterns of behavior began in the unconscious mind, they can be permanently changed at that level. This makes it possible to break the connection between your beliefs and your perceived inevitable outcome.

The unconscious mind is accessed through hypnosis, which is a naturally-occurring state of mind. In hypnosis, your focus of attention is narrowed and directed to your inner thought processes. It allows you to become aware of deeper aspects of your unconscious mind that can lead to the desired changes in your thoughts, feelings, beliefs and behaviors; in my case, to believe that cancer was not a death sentence and healing from it was possible.

How do these changes in thoughts, feelings, beliefs and behavior happen? They occur through what I call multi-sensory guided imagery, which is a focused relaxation to create harmony between your mind and body. Using the imagination to engage all of your senses helps to promote changes in your thoughts, feelings, beliefs and behaviors, thus encouraging emotional and physical healing. Through hypnosis with guided imagery, it is possible to disengage beliefs that interfere with your need and desire for something different, such as healing.

Many people think that they can't be hypnotized. The fact is that each of us goes in and out of light to medium states of hypnosis every day – many times a day.

Have you ever driven to work or to a friend's house and when you arrived, you didn't remember making all the turns or passing the familiar landmarks along the way? You were in hypnosis while your unconscious mind took over and performed the repetitive and familiar pattern of behavior. Perhaps when watching a scary movie, you felt your pulse racing when you thought the character was in great danger? What was happening in the movie was not real but your unconscious mind couldn't tell the difference.

One question I am often asked is, "What does it feel like to be hypnotized?" Some people don't feel radically different when they are hypnotized. Some people feel deeply relaxed and have a heavy feeling as if they were sinking into the chair. Other people may experience a lightness – a kind of floating or drifting sensation. And some people may experience a tingling sensation. *I'm a tingler. Very pleasant.*

Whatever you experience is exactly right for you. During hypnosis some people try to consciously listen to every word that is said. Others drift in and out of conscious awareness.

Still others do not hear much of anything that is said. Whether or not you were listening, whether or not you remember what was said doesn't matter because your unconscious mind takes it all in. Remember, your unconscious mind is capable of beginning to act on the suggestions without your needing to participate consciously during the session.

Now, if a suggestion were made that you found to be contrary to your morals or ethics, your conscious mind would override that suggestion. You cannot be made to do anything that you don't want to do, however, hypnosis can help you do something that you *do* want to do – like healing, or to stop smoking or lose weight, to name a few things.

There really is nothing scary about hypnosis. You simply relax and allow yourself to change your undesirable thoughts, feelings, beliefs or behaviors into positive, healthy and desirable thoughts, feelings, beliefs or behaviors. It is not magic. Anyone with a desire to change and offering no resistance to the process can be hypnotized. I teach all of my clients how to do self-hypnosis. It takes a little bit of practice but is well worth the effort.

I regularly use self-hypnosis at the dentist or to help me reach a quiet and reflective state of mind, for example. I also listen to hypnosis CD recordings like the one that I made for myself to listen to during my surgery. I enjoy being hypnotized by my hypnosis colleagues because it gives me a new perspective on whatever issue I am working on.

Chakra Balancing

Chakras are vortices in the body that represent centers of activity that are said to receive, express and assimilate Qi or life force energy and are responsible for how we function on a physical, emotional and spiritual level. There are seven major Chakras that correlate directly to the seven major endocrine glands of the body. The endocrine system is responsible for all of the physiological processes in our body. According to biologist Dr. Bruce Lipton, there is a direct link between our thoughts and emotions and their effect on our biology, indeed our DNA. In Sanskrit, Chakra means disk or wheel, and they are considered to be open or in balance when the energy is spinning in a clockwise direction. When our Chakras are out of balance, that is, the flow of energy is disrupted or blocked, there is a corresponding disruption in the balance and harmony of our physical, emotional and spiritual self.

While there are many Chakras in the body, for simplicity, I will just address the seven major and most familiar Chakras that align with the spine.

The first is the *Root Chakra* which is located in the perineum; the space between the anus and the scrotum or the vagina. It is connected to Gaia or Mother Earth and energetically represents our primitive survival and fear instincts. When this Chakra is open, we are grounded and connected to nature. The vibrational color for the Root Chakra is red.

The *Sacral Chakra* is the second Chakra and can be found four finger breadths below the umbilicus (belly button). It is referred to as the seat of our passions and houses our feelings and emotions energetically. It is the heart of our sense of worth, lovability and self-esteem and it is where our creativity resides. Anger closes us to abundant creative expression and romantic intimacy. The vibrational color for the Sacral Chakra is orange.

Third is the *Solar Plexus Chakra* found just below the xyphiod process or in layman's terms, below the bottom of the breast bone. The level of physical energy is located here. Maintaining the balance of this Chakra provides a high level of physical energy, helps good relationships with others to thrive and allows us clarity in the way we express ourselves. The vibrational color for the Solar Plexus Chakra is yellow.

The fourth is the *Heart Chakra* and is located at the center of the chest at about mid-sternum or the middle of the breast bone. This is the place where we experience unconditional love, compassion, and acceptance of everyone and everything in the universe. It is at the center of our physical energy system. When the Heart Chakra is closed, we are incapable of fully experiencing the joy of unconditional love, however, when it is open, we are also open to our greatest capacity for love and happiness. The vibrational color for the Heart Chakra is green.

Fifth in line is the *Throat Chakra* and can be found by locating the little "U" shape at the top of the breast bone, also referred to as the base of the throat. This, energetically, houses our verbal, nonverbal and psychic communication center for expressing our thoughts, feelings, ideas, hopes and dreams. When this Chakra is closed, we are unable to fully give "voice" to expressing ourselves. The vibrational color for the Throat Chakra is blue.

The sixth is the *Third Eye Chakra* located in the middle of the forehead. Known for being the keeper of our awareness, insight, vision, intuition, and focus, a closed Third Eye Chakra causes our awareness and focus to become clouded. The vibrational color for the Third Eye Chakra is deep indigo.

The seventh and last of the major Chakras is the *Crown Chakra*. It can be found at the very top of the head and is the portal to the heavens. It is our connection to our cosmic consciousness and enlightenment. It is where our divine purpose resides. When this Chakra is blocked, we may ask ourselves, "Is this all there is?" When it is open, we have a knowing that there is so much more for us to learn and to be. The vibrational colors for the Crown Chakra are violet to white.

Some areas that Chakra balancing may help with are mental clarity and awareness, deeper spiritual connections, decision making, energy, WellBeing, stress relief, love and sexual expression. Chakras can be balanced, opened or cleared in many different ways. A few methods are hypnosis, meditation, yoga, Reiki, guided imagery, reflexology and massage, to name just a few.

My friend Roxy combined Reiki, hypnosis and Chakra balancing in my pre-surgery session. I was able to achieve the most profoundly relaxing and calming state of mind that I have ever experienced. It allowed me to get more centered and focused while strengthening my newly-formed belief that complete healing was possible. All of my Chakras were so far out of whack, I am amazed that Roxy was able to get all of my vortices spinning in the right direction.

Bless you, Roxie!

CHAPTER TWENTY SEVEN

TOOLS

As with the techniques, this list is by no means comprehensive but reflects my personal experience.

Healing Recordings

There are many audio recordings available for different kinds of healing that employ a variety of techniques. By far, the most popular are hypnosis and meditation CDs. Some CDs are specific for things like stress relief, smoking cessation and weight loss. There are also some DVDs that feature visual imagery as well as sound. They can be found in abundance on the internet using search words such as healing, hypnosis, meditation, Chakra balancing, etc. Many practitioners produce their own recordings for generic healing or will customize one for your particular needs. You can also make your own, which takes a bit of techno savvy.

Music

Healing music is an essential element of healing as far as I am concerned. The three ingredients that I believe are the most important in choosing music are: first, it resonates with you – that is, that you find it pleasing to listen to;

second, it has a soothing tempo (60 beats per minute is optimal); and third, it is recorded at a frequency of 444Hz. Most recorded music is 440Hz and it is dissonant. The difference is striking when compared side by side. Music tuned to 444Hz is the secret chord that David played and it pleased the Lord. It is known as the Key of David. *See www.wholetones.com and learn more.*

Books

There is a huge array of books available for every kind of healing. They range from espousing radical changes in lifestyle and nutrition to religious, spiritual, motivational, transformational and inspirational. There is also a fair share of what many would consider to be out and out quackery. Years ago, I would have said all of the above fit into that category. You will find a lot of conflicting advice and information. Give it your due diligence and choose carefully. While the vast majority of books out there are written with good intentions, there are some hacks, charlatans and snake oil salesmen who prey on the sick just to make a buck. I like to think of it as a buffet. I take a little bit that resonates with me from each book. This is where your intuition and higher guidance comes in.

Crystals, Candles and Aromatherapy

This is a subject far too vast to adequately cover here so I am offering them as other avenues to explore to enhance your healing.

Crystals and gemstones are said to possess spiritual and healing properties that can be accessed in a variety of ways. Crystals may be kept near your body or worn as a piece of jewelry. They can also be placed on your body over an area where their healing vibrations are most needed or placed over your Chakras for balance. Each crystal has its own unique function and vibrational frequency. Their colors, shapes, and textures all have special significance. Water can be "charged" by soaking crystals using a glass pitcher. Healing crystals may be used for meditation. Use your intuition when picking out your crystal by choosing which one you are most attracted to.

I am fairly sensitive to certain crystals, meaning that I often feel tingling and warmth in my hands when holding them. I have collected a variety of crystals both large and small over the years mainly because I think they are beautiful and perhaps because I am drawn to them for their healing powers.

The flickering flame of a candle can be mesmerizing and quite soothing. A scented candle can be very pleasant as well. Candles are oftentimes used as a focal point for meditation. I prefer a campfire in the woods of Vermont, however, a candle is a safe and convenient substitute. I simply use my imagination to see the campfire.

The sense of smell is quite powerful and different scents can transport you to a happier time or remind you of a loved one. Choose any scent that pleases you.

Essential oils are purified oils extracted from natural plants and trees and are said to have many healing qualities. They are used topically, internally, as an inhalant or with a diffuser. An aroma therapist would be able to guide you as to what would be most beneficial to you. Some people use incense. I find that to be too strong but it definitely gives me a flashback to my hippie days.

CHAPTER TWENTY-EIGHT

TIPS

Screw the Stats

When it comes to survival statistics, stay away from Google. It will scare the crap out of you. Even if the stats indicate that there is a 1% chance of survival. Who says it won't be you? Why not you? Someone has to be in that 1%. If I had known the dismal stats for my prognosis, it would have really messed with my head. Being a nurse, I had a pretty good idea, however, I chose not to clutter my healing path by comparing my chances with how other people fared with the same diagnosis. Stats are just numbers that have nothing to do with you as an individual and your ability to self-heal. Screw the stats and skew the curve.

Good Humor

Humor is good for what ails you, especially when you're really "crabby" (pun intended). A sense of humor will hold you in good stead. Laughter has an extremely positive effect on you both physiologically and emotionally; however, I would recommend laying off the belly laughs after major abdominal surgery so you don't bust a gut. Otherwise, I think it's a great way to release tension and reduce stress. Get your chuckles anywhere you can, watching YouTube videos, funny movies, just being goofy or reading a good book about healing cancer.

Stop Smoking

If you are a smoker, there is one thing that will absolutely contribute to your healing and that is to **STOP SMOKING!** Don't wait until you are faced with a serious illness. Now is always the best time to quit. Having been a two pack-a-day smoker, I know from whence I speak and I am passionate about helping people **STOP SMOKING.** After your last cigarette, your body immediately begins to repair the damage from smoking and will speed your healing in general.

Lose Some Attitude and Choose Some Gratitude

There is not a day that goes by that I am not grateful for something. I am grateful for most things in my life and for some things that are not in my life anymore, like cancer. I endeavor to practice giving thanks every day although some days are easier than others. Sometimes I need a nudge and a gentle reminder from my friends, family and colleagues. Gratitude is high up in the Green Zone of your emotional hierarchy and it is an essential part of WellBeing, making it a prime ingredient for healing. Feeling and expressing gratitude is an excellent way to raise your vibrational frequency.

There are many ways to practice gratitude and the choice is yours. Some keep a gratitude journal. That's just not for me. I don't think I have the discipline for that. Others make lists. I like lists but I don't take the time to write things down on a consistent basis.

What I like to do is to review my day before I fall asleep at night. I focus on the good and fun things that happened during the day. I also think about what I will do the next day that will bring me joy – even a tiny bit of it. I don't necessarily call it a gratitude exercise, but it works for me. It was not always easy to find things that made me feel grateful. It took a little practice and now it is a habit.

I like to play a little game that I call "But at least I..." Whenever something unpleasant or upsetting happens, I find some reason to balance it out with something good that happened. For example, I got cancer but at least I healed myself. It really works especially when several unexpectedly upsetting events pile up or are bunched in a group. I had a week about ten years ago that was just one giant cluster f**k. My little game saved me from going completely over the edge. It went like this:

I injured my arm but at least it wasn't broken.

When I left the doctor's office, I had a flat tire but at least I had a spare.

The tire was shot but at least the mechanic could put a new one on that same day.

The mechanic backed his truck into my car and creamed it pretty good but at least he said he would fix it and rent me a car.

My car insurance was cancelled because I forgot to send in a survey (Do you believe that?) and I couldn't rent a car in my name but at least I was able to use a friend's car.

I rear-ended a car at a red light with my friend's car but at least *she* had insurance.

My car insurance tripled after the cancellation but at least I had the money to pay it.

My driver's license was revoked because my car insurance was cancelled but at least my car was fixed.

I got my license back and then got a speeding ticket but at least I didn't get any points (I hired a lawyer).

I was at my wits' end and complaining bitterly to a friend about my awful week and she said, "But at least it's not cancer."

So many people think that cancer is the yardstick by which all bad things are measured. I used to think so too. While I can't say that I am actually grateful for having had cancer, I am grateful for the blessings I have received because of it.

In this episode of my life, some of the things for which I am grateful are that I was healed and didn't die, though I had plenty of close calls, my mother is at peace, I had a wonderful WellBeing Team that supported me throughout, and I have a new found way of being and a clear purpose for being here.

Journey to Joy

The journey to joy is complex. It is at the very top of the Green Zone. Anger is the one thing that will stop you in your tracks on your way to joyfulness. Anger takes many forms, sometimes obvious and other times hidden. Nothing keeps you as stuck in the Red Zone as holding on to your anger. Joy can only exist in the presence of peace. There can be no peace in the presence of anger. There can be no anger in the presence of forgiveness so it follows, then, without forgiveness, you will remain *stuck* without any hope of the joyful life you so richly deserve. Letting go of anger is not easy and it is a difficult job to do alone. Seek out an EFT practitioner or a therapist to help you. There are certainly other helpful modalities but this is my preferred route.

Forgiving Family, Friends, and Foe

Keep this in mind: you must forgive for your own sake, for your own peace of mind. The thing about forgiveness is that it is for your benefit. It is a selfish act and that is okay. The recipient of your forgiveness does not even have to know it, they may not want it or need it and they may not really care. It is all about using that negative energy, wasted on another, and turning it into positive energy to be used for your highest good. When you are able to forgive, you are no longer giving away your power but rather taking it back.

Do this little forgiveness exercise using some very powerful "I am" statements. To begin the process of forgiving, think of someone who has caused you to feel angry, someone for whom you are holding a grudge, someone with whom you can't get past being angry. They can be alive or passed. It might even be yourself that needs forgiveness. Now decide that you are willing to forgive them. Make a commitment to forgive them. The relief and release you feel will be well worth your effort. Forgive one person at a time and repeat these statements until you feel the truth in your heart.

I am acknowledging that forgiveness is the key to my peace of mind.

I am acknowledging that forgiveness is difficult to do.

I am acknowledging that forgiveness is possible to do.

I am acknowledging that forgiveness is necessary to do.

I am acknowledging that forgiveness is the right thing to do.

I am acknowledging that forgiveness is the kindest thing to do.

I am acknowledging that forgiveness is the loving thing to do.

I am willing to forgive those who have angered me.

I am willing to forgive those who have saddened me.

I am willing to forgive those who have hurt me.

I am willing to forgive those who have abandoned me.

I am willing to forgive those who have betrayed me.

I am willing to forgive those who have been disloyal to me.

I am willing to forgive those who have treated me unfairly.

I am willing to forgive for my own sake.

Get Out of My Head

Did you ever get a song stuck in your head and you just couldn't get it out? You know, some stupid jingle or the last song you heard on the radio before you left your car to go in to work. This happened to me a lot during my stint in the healthcare system. No, I did not get a song stuck in my head but I got a daily barrage of unintentionally thoughtless and insensitive comments and explanations meant to inform me of unwanted details about my health status.

One only need start with this little ditty, "a clot could break off and go to your heart, your lungs or your brain and kill you." Then there's the hematology fellow who told me that I was "cancer free...for now." After having a second post-op CA125 drawn for my six-month follow-up Gyn/Onc visit, the nurse told me that the level was fifteen. "Good for me," I exclaimed. It was well within the normal range. Then she said, "It's creeping up." I mentioned that I had a long way to go before it got to 17,000. She meant no harm by it but it got in my head just the same. When Dr. Grace came in and joyfully shared the results of the CA125, I said, "Yeah, but it's creeping up." Even though Dr. Grace laughed it off as we shared what she thought was a little joke, it still stuck in my head. I had to work really hard to get that one out.

I had become acutely aware of the things that got stuck in my head and it made me angry. This was actually a good thing because I was aware and could deal with it head-on in the moment. When I shared the whole "stuck in your head" thing with a group of caregivers, they wondered why it was better to recognize it because if you didn't notice it, it couldn't bother you. Wrong! For every ditty I caught flying in, there were a hundred that came in under the radar. They went unnoticed but still were doing their damage nonetheless.

If something doesn't sit well or feel quite right, deal with it. Talk it out. Do whatever you need to do to make it okay. I may be sounding like a broken record, however, EFT works wonders with stuck stuff too.

Navigating Shark-Infested Waters

You have got to stand up for yourself when dealing with the healthcare system. It can be a bit like navigating shark-infested waters. After my first visit with Dr. Grace, I couldn't think straight. The next thing I knew, I was being set up for more scans, more blood work and being put on the OR schedule. My life had been taken over by strangers. I felt overwhelmed and out of control.

Nothing in my forty years as a nurse ever prepared me for being on the receiving end of this kind of news. I needed to be a full participant in my own healing. After all, it was *my* body. I needed a little breathing room. As much as I wanted the cancer out of my body *right now,* it was essential for me to step back and get on top of the fear, allowing me to make some rational decisions after exploring *all* of my treatment options before I committed to anything.

After the first two hospitalizations dealing with the blood clots, I decided that I had to be true to myself. I was no longer willing to lie down and play dead. No one was going to ride roughshod over me. When I made my needs and my intentions clear, it was not a problem. And if it was, I dealt with it.

I have been told that it must have been easier for me to stand up for myself because I am a nurse. Yes and no. I have more medical knowledge than the average patient, however, my issues were not in my field of expertise. Even when the patient may be a doctor or a nurse, they are, first and foremost, the patient; that is, they have the same fears and concerns as any other patient. We were taught never to make assumptions about what a patient does and does not know even if they have a medical background. I had as many questions as any other patient and perhaps more.

My advice is to make your needs and intentions clear to everyone who comes in contact with you. Do not be afraid to ask questions, to get clarification and to have things "dumbed down" for you. I did, plenty of times. Don't worry about taking up too much of the nurse's or doctor's time. They work for you! Channel your inner two year old and keep asking "Why?" until you are satisfied with the answers.

A Word about Nutrition

Discussion of the role of nutrition in my healing has been conspicuously absent. There are two reasons for this, the first being that I believed with so little time before surgery, radical dietary changes would have been of little benefit on the immediate outcome. The second reason is that I could not do justice to the vast topic of nutrition with so many other excellent resources available to guide you.

Your WellBeing Team

Quite by accident, I began assembling my Pep Squad as each person showed up with unwavering and unconditional support of my declaration to be well. Even when I faltered, they remained steadfast. Many more friends and colleagues have been added over time and I am grateful for each one of them. The name of the team has changed over time from my Pep Squad to my Healing Team to my WellBeing Team, opting to keep the focus on the wellness and not the illness.

Who should you have on your WellBeing Team? Even if you are in tiptop shape, it is always a good idea to be surrounded with supportive, caring, loving, kick-you-in-the-ass-when-you-need-it kind of folks. They can be family, friends, colleagues, healthcare professionals, coaches, mentors, clergy and holistic arts practitioners. This group may ebb and flow or increase or decrease in the number of members as needed.

This may be my own bias, however, every WellBeing Team should have a nurse on it. It is best if she (or he) has a leaning toward integrating the holistic alternative healing arts. Everyone knows a nurse or knows someone who knows a nurse. Nurses are always willing to answer a question or talk about general wellness practices and guide you in the right direction for additional care. There are many nurses who have integrated CAM modalities into their nursing practice, bringing you the best of both worlds. Some offer their services in a private practice setting as I do. Just keep in mind that a nurse cannot make a diagnosis or treat an ailment without a physician's or an Advanced Nurse Practitioner's order.

Who should not be on your WellBeing Team? The important thing is to shield yourself from naysayers, toxic people, emotional vampires, reality checkers, devil's advocates and the loving saboteurs. These folks will take up residence in your head. You won't always know them when you see them, so beware. Listen to your WellBeing Team if they see any red flags you might have missed.

Keep your eyes, mind and heart open for potential team members because you never know how or when they will show up. You can be sure of one thing, though, they will show up!

CHAPTER TWENTY-NINE

TRICK OR TREAT?

Earlier, I had mentioned that shortly after hearing the results of the special MRI, I popped a couple of bite-size Snickers before going to bed. The whole truth is that Snickers soon became my mainstay diet up until I was hospitalized in preparation for the surgery. As was my usual morning routine, I started my day with a nice healthy protein shake. Generally speaking, my resolve for healthy eating would quickly dissolve as the day wore on, however, the Snickers thing was a completely new wrinkle. After my shake, I snacked on those mini bites throughout the day, often skipping lunch and sometimes supper too. I ate them by the bagful.

I didn't question myself about this nor was I particularly concerned about it. I wanted those little Snickers. In fact, I had an unrelenting craving for them. I gave in without putting up even a smidgeon of resistance. Sometime later, I asked myself why I did this. On some level, I realized that I needed a treat, a reward or some sort of comfort food. Why Snickers? Other than Snickers bars having been the prized score on Halloween as a child, I hadn't a clue. I just went with it. I also thought that on the off chance that I might croak, I was going to go out in a blaze of chocolate! Interestingly, after surgery, Snickers were no longer my go-to sweet treat.

For the first couple of years after healing, I had difficulty wrapping my head around the enormity of the amazing blessing and precious gift I had received. Sometimes I would ponder the extremely thoughtless comments some clueless people made to me that perhaps they missed some of the cancer and it would come roaring back. I could usually push them away, which sometimes took a considerable amount of effort.

Approaching the two-year mark (I prefer not to commemorate it as an anniversary) after surgery, I had some slight trepidation about my upcoming checkup with Dr. Grace. It was not all-consuming but rather was an ever-present lurking under the surface. The night before my appointment, I had a dream that I was in the stairwell of the hospital. I was not sure why I was there when suddenly Dr. Grace came trotting down the stairs wearing her lab coat and carrying a clipboard. "Why aren't you upstairs? They are waiting for you!"

"Waiting for me? Why?"

"You're scheduled for your chemo today."

"No, no, no! I was healed. Remember? You told me there was nothing there to treat."

Furiously leafing through the pages on her clipboard, she stopped at the last page, looked up at me with a smile and said, "Oh, that's right, you already had the Snickers Therapy!"

I took that as a positive sign that all was well and it was.

CHAPTER THIRTY

DYING TO BE HEALED

There were times when I pondered just how fragile my physical self had become and I realized that this cancer could have put an end to my mortal existence in a skip of a heartbeat. Not to sound morbid or fatalistic but it was a statistical possibility. Good thing I chose to embrace the sentiments of my friend, Roxy who said, "F**k the facts and f**k the cancer too!" *Words to live by.*

To get to a place of fearlessness, I had to consider death as a potential reality and not just in the abstract. Getting a cancer diagnosis made my mind take a straight shot from cancer to fear to pain to death in a nanosecond. I came to know that, ultimately, it was not death that I feared as much as the actual process of dying.

When I was a freshman in nursing school, part of our training was to shadow a visiting nurse for a day. One visit became permanently etched in my memory. A woman in her early forties (my mother's age) with three young children was in the terminal stages of colon cancer. Weak and frail, her body had been ravaged beyond my comprehension. Her face was contorted and her body wrenched uncontrollably as she begged her husband to stop the pain. He stood helplessly by, unable to give her any comfort because she had been given the maximum amount of pain medication that the doctor ordered. She would have to wait another hour for her next dose.

The visiting nurse said she would call the doctor when she got back to the office (many hours later) and see if he could order something stronger (knowing that he would not). The call to the doctor was unnecessary as this poor woman blessedly passed away within an hour of our visit. This was more than forty years ago and hospice was not a widely available option. Effective pain management was nonexistent, as it was feared that a patient might get addicted to the narcotics or an overdose might suppress their respirations and hasten their death even though they were dying.

I was eighteen years old and I was not prepared for anything like this. I was so shaken and horrified by this experience that I vowed that I would never allow someone that I cared for to suffer like that and for sure, not me either. Sadly, there were many times in my career that I could not keep that promise to a patient who, clutching my hand with superhuman strength, begged me to end their suffering. The look in their eyes pierced my soul and haunts me to this day.

This chapter was not on my radar as I began the final edit of this book. The book had to take a back seat for a while so I could help The Other Pat care for her cousin, Kathy, who was in the end stages of lung cancer with metastasis to the bone, liver and brain and could no longer care for herself. Her immediate family was all gone. She had a few cousins and a small network of friends. I did not know Kathy well, however, I did know that she had many health challenges throughout her life, including two strokes and epilepsy, yet remained fiercely and stubbornly independent.

Kathy was first diagnosed in September of 2011 at the age of fifty-five. She had been saying for the past several months that she was ready to die. She did not want any more chemo or radiation. She wanted to be with her parents, her sister and her cats. During a recent visit with Kathy, I admired several antique pieces she had and she shared the stories of her "garbage picking" adventures. I stopped commenting on her things when she offered to let me to take anything that I admired home with me. It turned out that during the last few weeks she had been giving away photos, record albums and other mementos to her closest friends.

Later in the visit when Pat went out to pick up lunch, Kathy shared with me that she was going to ask the doctor to put her to sleep. She was not afraid of dying but she did not want to die alone. I asked what she was waiting for and she told me some people were not ready to let her go. I told her that some people will never be ready and that it would be all right for her to just let go.

Shortly after that visit, the effects of the cancer in her brain made it impossible for Kathy to live by herself any longer. I was happy to help Pat care for Kathy. It allowed me to pay it forward for all the care and support Pat had given me during my healing process. I must admit that I had some trepidation about being so intimately involved in the final leg of Kathy's journey. I was reminded of the phrase I so often heard as a child, "There but for the grace of God go I."

It was Saturday, November 15, 2014 when Pat took over Kathy's care. She was extremely weak, had no appetite and was having intermittent abdominal pain which was relieved by her pain pills. Despite being a little fuzzy about time and place, she talked easily about her childhood memories of family vacations at the lake and of the fun the cousins had growing up. She talked about where she had travelled and of her different jobs. This is called the life review. I knew that this, along with giving away her worldly possessions, meant the end was not far away. By the next day she stopped eating and grew weaker still. She was unable to hold a conversation of any substance with us; however, she had begun to have some rather animated conversations with her parents, her sister, her grandmother and her cats, who appeared to be hovering in an upper corner of her room.

Pat, my sister Jean and I had taken turns staying up at night with Kathy and an odd thing happened during my shift on Monday night. As I was walking Kathy to the bathroom, I glanced at the digital clock on the DVR to see what time it was. I could not see the display clearly but it looked like letters and not numbers. When I got closer, the display clearly read "pRaY". Pray? I did a double take and watched as the word changed back to three-fifteen a.m. I was a little freaked out but not frightened. I wondered why I needed a reminder to pray. Although no longer being tethered to a particular faith, I still have informal communication with Source. If that is considered prayer, then what I was praying for was for Kathy to be free of pain and at peace. I thought about the significance of three-fifteen a.m. It is often referred to as the "Witching Hour" or the "Devil's Time". For me, awakening at three-fifteen, as I frequently do, is usually when I have moments of great clarity.

I was concerned that her pain management would be inadequate given my previous student nurse experience and as a pediatric hospice nurse in the '90s. It took about twenty-four hours for Kathy to get complete relief. In addition to the pain, she had what is called terminal restlessness, which made her a bit combative when it came to taking the medication or rendering care. By Thursday she was comfortable with occasional restlessness. Friday afternoon her body was completely relaxed and she was in what appeared to be a comatose state. On Saturday, 11/22 at 11:22 a.m., Kathy sighed and peacefully, took her final breath. She was not alone and was free of pain just as she had wanted.

Some might wonder why I would include a story about someone who died from cancer in a book about healing from cancer. I was on the fence about this for some time and the simple truth is that, sadly, some people are going to die from cancer. The fact is that we are all going to die from something at some point.

I have come to believe that healing does not always mean physical healing. Sometimes healing happens on a soul level, not on a conscious level. For Kathy, I believe that her soul decision was to find peace and to be with her family. When a loved one dies, look past the failure of the physical body to heal and rejoice in the freedom of their spirit.

In going through this process with Kathy, I learned that it wasn't about not wanting to die but rather wanting to live. I had things to do, places to go and people to see. I knew I had been kept around for a reason. I want and need and am driven to share a message with as much of the world as I can reach, that healing from cancer (or any illness) is possible if that is your soul's desire. Understand that a soul decision is not necessarily a conscious choice to let go. It is not a death wish.

So, for me, it is the suffering and not death that was my greatest fear. As for dying, while I am in no hurry, I know there will be an amazing new soul adventure in store for me and when I decide to come back for another visit to this earthly plane, I will be richer, smarter and thinner.

CHAPTER THIRTY-ONE

WORLDS COLLIDING

For the past twenty years, I had been living with one foot in the world of alternative healing, a burgeoning spirituality and an ever-expanding "energy" awareness, while the other foot was firmly planted in the world of everyday conventional, take-a-pill-for-whatever-ails-you existence. In recent years, the people with whom I frequently came in contact were of the same metaphysical ilk. Among them were colleagues, clients and mentors. It took some adjustment to accommodate this duality. I worried, as George Costanza from *Seinfeld* did, that my worlds would collide if I hosted a social gathering that included both my "real life" friends and my "woo-woo" friends. It did happen on my sixtieth birthday, but there were was no colliding of my worlds. Just my good friends enjoying a meal together. During my frequent health visits and hospitalizations, however, the collisions became routine. The expectation of the healthcare traditionalists was that I would be a compliant and acquiescent patient, drinking the Kool-Aid and taking the party line where my care and treatment was concerned. *Not so much.*

My "real life" friends are unwaveringly supportive of me even though some of them don't get that other side of me. The "me" who was a patient who happened to be a nurse did not always feel that support with the exception a precious few. Of course, Dr. Grace was at the top of that very short list. I am not complaining...anymore, although I did my share of whining about it during the temporary disruption in my otherwise robust health back in '09.

In my professional life, I completely stepped away from traditional nursing in 2009 P.C. (post crabs), and I no longer feel like I have a foot in each of two worlds anymore. In fact, it doesn't feel like there are two worlds at all. I am comfortable with who I am being now and I am more tolerant of and gentle with those who have not yet, as I jokingly say, come over to the light side.

CHAPTER THIRTY-TWO

LESSONS ALONG THE WAY

Ultimately, this book was not about cancer. *Say what?* Okay, so there was a lot about cancer in it, but it really serves as a backdrop to showcase what we are capable of accomplishing; that is, extraordinary healing. It could have been about any catastrophic illness or event. For me, it just happened to be cancer and let's face it, cancer definitely gets your attention. It's always been about the healing and not the cancer.

Let's Review

I wanted to share with you some things I learned and to review some other things. In no particular, order, let's begin with the Healing Triad. One, get a handle on your fear. Two, SPEAK UP! You must speak up for yourself as loudly as possible so you can get what you want and what you need. Three, overhaul your entire belief system by giving those worn out and useless beliefs that do more harm than good the old heave-ho and replace them with bright shiny new ones that you can live with...literally.

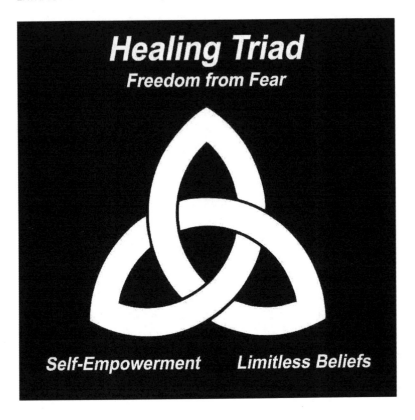

Resistance is Futile

I always intended to mention this but I never found the right place so I'm sticking it in here. *Better late than never.* Resistance is like a gremlin that lives in our head. We are programmed to resist change. We thrive on sameness. Not because we like to be bored but because sameness is comfortable. It is familiar and expected. It only becomes an issue when things change around us or inside of us that we resist making the necessary adjustments, physically or emotionally, to accommodate it or get rid of it. It is in our nature to resist change but so is learning to adapt a part of our nature.

Abraham-Hicks uses the metaphor of a canoe in a stream. If your canoe is facing downstream, you must paddle backwards with all of your might to resist the flow of the current just to stay where you are. If you take your paddle out of the water and go with the flow, the resistance is gone. This does not mean that you are going with the flow of the cancer, it simply means that you are letting go of the struggle, allowing you to find another solution.

You may need to make uncomfortable changes in your life which require making some uncomfortable decisions. That could mean changing or quitting your job in pursuit of reclaiming your WellBeing. I did not go back to my soul-sucking job after reclaiming my WellBeing because it was not in my highest good. It wasn't great for me financially but is was the right thing for me to do. There may be some toxic relationships that need to change or end. You will need to get rid of the naysayers, enablers and emotional vampires to give your life some peace. I didn't fire any friends outright, however, some I allowed to drift away without feeling guilty about not reconnecting.

Nothing will ever be the same in your life after cancer as it was before. Just remember that different is not necessarily a bad thing. Everyone assumes that when the treatment is finished or your WellBeing is reclaimed, you will just pick up where you left off. It is not the end. It is a new and different beginning.

Ask and You Shall Receive

There is no need to walk your path alone. There are some people who will be by your side every step of the way. *Just be sure you want them there.* There are others who will walk at least part of the journey with you. Some you know and others you have yet to meet. People and things will show up when you need them most. You just have to learn to recognize them when they do show up. You must ask for whom or what you need. I did not feel comfortable asking anyone to walk my path with me. It turns out that I didn't have to ask. They were always there and they walked along with me willingly.

I had no plan when I started on my healing path. I knew what I wanted and left it up to the Universe to light my way. I had to be open and alert to recognize what I needed when it crossed my path. If something showed up unexpectedly, I had to discard the notion that it was a coincidence or a random find and embrace it. It took a little practice but then I got really good at it. The more I opened up, the more I found. The truth is that it was there all along, I just never saw it before because I never needed to look for it before.

Clear Your Emotional Clutter

If you have chosen to pursue a holistic approach to your healing, begin by finding a practitioner to help you clear away all of your negative crap. There are many modalities to choose from. I have listed the ones that were helpful to me in Chapter 26 and I have listed others in the Recommendations and Resources that may also be helpful. Insurance does not generally pay for this kind of healing. For those of you who care about someone with cancer and feel helpless but want to do something, why not give them a holistic healing shower with healing sessions as gifts. *Wish I'd thought of that sooner.*

Celebrate WellBeing

The most important thing that I want to share with you is to remember to always celebrate your WellBeing. I know it is not always easy. Many times along the way, it was the farthest thing from my mind. When you look at the checks and balances of your life, it is easy to see what's in the minus column. We tend to take for granted the many blessings in the plus column.

I have talked a lot about things needing to be in balance. I like things to be balanced. I have a compulsive need for bilateral symmetry. If I put a couch in the room, there must be identical end tables on either side of it. *I'm working on that.* When it comes to WellBeing vs. all the crap, I am all for tipping the scales in favor of a celebration.

Wrapping It Up

So that's it. My whole story. I had no other agenda in writing this book other than to share my experience and hope others touched by cancer could glean some benefit from it. I don't know what the takeaway will be for you, but no matter where you or a loved one are on your healing odyssey – the beginning, somewhere in the middle or nearing the finish line (and I don't mean death) – my hope is that you will be inspired, emboldened, empowered and secure in your belief that an ordinary miracle is possible for your extraordinary healing.

Now go celebrate your WellBeing!

EPILOGUE

It's been nearly six years since my healing odyssey began and I am frequently asked, "How are you doing now?" meaning since the cancer. The simple answer is, "Fine, thanks, and you?" A more meaningful question that would yield a more meaningful response would be to query, "How are you *being* now?" *Again with the semantics.* If you have discovered anything about me in this book, it is that language plays an important role in every aspect of my being.

I am forever changed. And I am not finished changing who I am being and I doubt that I ever will be. So who am I being right now? Exactly who I was meant to be right in this very moment. Okay, this is beginning to sound a bit esoteric and is a perfect example of how worlds can collide. I didn't always understand the subtleties of what I refer to as *spirit speak* or *metaphysicalese*. Who you are being instead of how you are doing is so much more than a matter of semantics.

Let me break it down a little. Ontology (not to be confused with oncology) is the study of being. Of being what? The Latin word, *esse* means "to be" and is the root word for essence and essential. So *being* means the essential nature or essence of a person. *Quiddity* is that certain je ne sais quoi or inherent and distinctive peculiarity of a person. It is the thing that makes you uniquely *you.*

Uddalaka Aruni, a philosopher whose teachings are recorded in the Hindu Upanishads (records of truth and ultimate reality) is quoted as saying, "There is an invisible essence from which all things evolve." Every experience in life changes us in some way and becomes part of our essence, sometimes dramatically and sometimes imperceptibly.

So what do I say when asked, "How are you doing?" For right now, I say, "I am being well with a whole lot of quiddity. Thanks for asking."

WHO IS NURSE CRILLY?

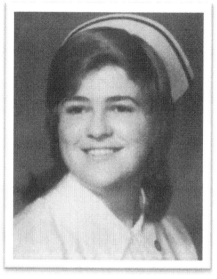

Patricia French Crilly, affectionately known to her colleagues and clients as Nurse Crilly, has been a Registered Nurse since 1973. In the mid-1990s, she began integrating the Holistic Alternative Healing Arts with nursing bringing a unique skillset to her current practice as a WellBeing Nurse Navigator. Nurse Crilly assists her clients in identifying and achieving their personal goals for healing the mind, body and spirit through Self-Directed Wellbeing by bridging the gap between allopathic medicine and holistic healing.

Nurse Crilly is certified as an Advanced Clinical Hypnotherapist, a Stress Management Consultant, a Trinfinity8 Practitioner and an EFT Practitioner and Trainer. In addition to *Extraordinary Healing, Ordinary Miracle*, Patricia is the author of *Tap It and Zap It! A Grownup's Guide to EFT for Kids* and has hosted her own radio show, *B-Positive with Nurse Crilly*.

Diagnosed with invasive ovarian and uterine cancer in 2009, Nurse Crilly set about finding a way to be completely healed without the need for extensive cancer treatment. Combining her skills as a nurse and as a practitioner of several holistic alternative healing modalities, she experienced what many declared to be a complete and miraculous healing. She knows that her extraordinary healing was indeed a miracle, an ordinary miracle that we are all capable of achieving and receiving.

Fulfilling her mission to help others for more than forty years as a nurse, her journey to WellBeing revealed her new mission. With equal doses of humor and compassion, she now shares her story from a diagnosis that paralyzed her with fear to changing her self-limiting belief that cancer is a death sentence and empowering herself to reclaim her WellBeing against tremendous odds. After a long and satisfying career in traditional nursing and recently declaring "been there, done that", Nurse Crilly is excited to pursue this new journey with her usual gusto and vigor.

Patricia also designs and conducts informative and inspiring workshops and seminars for the general public, corporations and health care professionals including: *Celebrate Your WellBeing, Navigating the Shark Infested Waters of the Health Care System, Integrating Holistic Healing Arts into Your Self-Care Regimen* and *WARNING! Medical Speak May Be Hazardous to Your Health.*

Nurse Crilly is available for Workshops, Seminars and Keynotes tailored for your organization or group. Contact her for more information about speaking or a bulk order for her book: info@ExtraordinaryHealingOrdinaryMiracle.com or call 732-339-1414.

RECOMMENDATIONS
AND RESOURCES

Techniques and Tools

Following are potentially helpful techniques and tools not mentioned earlier in this book. Some of them were unavailable to me or I was unaware of them during the time of my Healing Odyssey. There are many hundreds of others, however, I am only listing those for which I have been certified or have personally experienced.

Healing Touch

Healing Touch is a relaxing, nurturing energy therapy that uses gentle touch to assist in balancing physical, mental, emotional and spiritual well-being. Healing Touch works with your energy field to support your natural ability to heal, is safe for all ages and works in harmony with standard or allopathic medical care.

To learn more, go to:
www.HealingBeyondBorders.org

Matrix Reimprinting

Matrix Reimprinting, using EFT, is a method to clear adverse feelings, negative learnings and painful past events. Like its predecessors, Matrix Reimprinting also uses the Traditional Chinese Medicine meridian system that has been used in acupuncture for thousands of years.

To learn more, go to: **www.MatrixReimprintingus.com**

Sedona Method

The Sedona Method is a simple, powerful, easy-to-learn technique that uncovers your natural ability to let go of uncomfortable emotions in the present. By asking yourself a series of questions leads your awareness to what you are feeling in the moment and gently guides you into the experience of letting go.

To learn more, go to: **www.Sedona.com**

Trinfinity8

Trinfinity8 represents a new quantum shift in the emerging science of algorithmic rejuvenation technology. The Trinfinity8 with its unique software program uses a personal computer to deliver non-invasive rejuvenation programs based on mathematical codes, vibrational energies, and fractal formulations that are in harmony with core energetics that encompass all of nature.

To learn more, go to:
www.YourRejuvenationStation.com

Stop Smoking

There are any number of methods available to help you or a loved one to stop smoking. I have developed a DIY Stop Smoking First Aid Kit designed to use in the privacy of your own home.

To learn more, go to: **www.ButtEnders.com**

Books

There are hundreds more to choose from. These are the top ten that resonated the most for me.

Ask and It is Given by Abraham-Hicks

The Vortex by Abraham-Hicks

Radical Remission by Kelly Turner, Ph.D.

Mind Over Medicine by Lissa Rankin, M.D.

The Biology of Belief by Bruce Lipton, Ph.D.

The Genie in Your Genes by Dawson Church, Ph.D.

Energy Medicine by Donna Eden

The Sound of Healing by Michael S. Tyrell

The Power of Intention by Dr. Wayne W. Dyer

Power vs. Force by David R. Hawkins M.D., Ph.D.

DVDs

The Science of Miracles by Gregg Braden (Features the woman with the inoperable bladder tumor melting away)

You Can Heal Your Life by Louise Hay

The Law of Attraction in Action by Abraham-Hicks (12 DVD set)

Music

Ordinary Miracles from the CD The Music Never Ends by Maureen McGovern. For more music, go to: **www.MaureenMcGovern.com**

Holy Harmony by Jonathan Goldman (*Features all of the Solfeggio Healing Frequencies*). For more music, go to: **www.HealingSounds.com**

237

Musical Massage by Janalea Hoffman. For more music, go to: **www.RythmicMedicine.com**

What Would You Do this Year If You Had No Fear? by Jana Stanfield. For more music, go to: **www.JanaStanfield.com**

Wholetones: The Healing Frequency Music Project by Michael S. Tyrrell.

To learn more, go to: **www.wholetones.com**

The path I forged to healing was vastly different than most people diagnosed with cancer take. My hope is to begin a ground swell to create a paradigm shift in how modern medicine and society treat, think and talk about healing from cancer. I am passionate about the message of hope and healing that I have to share and I can't think of a better way to start than for you to write a review of my book and to begin talking, blogging and tweeting about it with friends, family and anyone whose life has been touched by cancer.

Please begin to share by going to:
www.bitly.com/reviewmybook **on Amazon.**
Thank you!

www.ExtraordinaryHealingOrdinaryMiracle.com

.

Made in the USA
Lexington, KY
16 July 2016